RUNNING UP THAT HILL

The Highs and Lows of Going That Bit Further

VASSOS ALEXANDER

BLOOMSBURY SPORT

LONDON · OXFORD · NEW YORK · NEW DELHI · SYDNEY

BLOOMSBURY SPORT
Bloomsbury Publishing Plc

50 Bedford Square, London, WC1B 3DP, UK

BLOOMSBURY, BLOOMSBURY SPORT and the Diana logo are trademarks of
Bloomsbury Publishing Plc

First published in Great Britain 2018
This edition published 2019

A catalogue record for this book is available from the British Library

Library of Congress Cataloguing-in-Publication data has been applied for

ISBN: PB: 978-1-4729-4795-6; eBook: 978-1-4729-4797-0

2 4 6 8 10 9 7 5 3 1

Typeset in Chaparral Pro by Deanta Global Publishing Services, Chennai, India
Printed and bound by CPI Group (UK) Ltd, Croydon, CR0 4YY

To find out more about our authors and books visit www.bloomsbury.com
and sign up for our newsletters

Running, life, the following races and pages … they're all about the journey, not the destination.
This book is for Caroline, Emily, Matthew and Mary.
Who are both.

acknowledgements

The one thing I've discovered about endurance runners – they're all so nice! It seems to go with the miles. So loads of ace people to thank.

First to everyone I've met along the trail, thank you for being so friendly and welcoming. I'm relatively new to this, not brilliant and not terrible, but really keen and utterly hooked; I hope the following pages will do your sport justice. It's the only reason I've written them.

My sincere gratitude to the many kind folk who agreed to be interviewed for this, all massively impressive runners who generously gave up their time. In order of appearance, thank you to Scott Jurek, Jasmin Paris, Nicky Spinks, Jez Bragg, Marcus Scotney, Dean Karnazes, Emelie Forsberg, Kilian Jornet, Debbie Martin-Consani, James Elson, Mimi Anderson, Dave Urwin, Nathan Flear, Elise Downing, Ben Smith, Julian Hall, Karl Meltzer, Charlie Engle and Claire Maxted. It was a proper privilege to speak to each and every one of you. Also, to the inspirational Chantel Scherer who's so knowledgeable about sports volunteering.

To the excellent team at Bloomsbury: Charlotte, Sarah, Zoë, Katherine, Lizzy and Alice, thank you for being brilliant (again).

Pheidippides probably deserves a mention too. Everyone who's ever run a marathon has the Ancient Greek messenger to thank for it. As do all of us lucky enough to have attempted the Spartathlon.

And lastly, mostly, to my wonderful family: to Caroline, Emily, Matthew and Mary – thank you for putting up with me disappearing on yet another long run. I do love running, but I love you much, much more.

8 May 2017 at 12:15
Email from: Chrissie Wellington
Subject: What have I done?!

Just entered!!!!!!!

8 May 2017 at 12:40
Reply from: Vassos Alexander
Re: What have I done?!

Hooray!! I promise you'll love it.

8 May 2017 at 12:46
Reply from: Chrissie Wellington
Re: What have I done?!

I
HATE
YOU

8 May 2017 at 15:40
Reply from: Vassos Alexander
Re: What have I done?!

Ha! See how much you hate me when you reach mile 44!!

I may have been mildly to blame for Chrissie entering her first ultra-marathon. Only in that I introduced her to the organiser and kept bombarding them both with emails until she agreed to give it a go. Still, she thanks me for it now. I think.

foreword

'I'LL. NEVER. DO. AN. ULTRA.'

I remember speaking to Vassos after he completed Race to the Stones and being sent a decidedly unattractive picture of his feet with their dead toenails and Vesuvius-sized blisters and swore I would never do an ultra-marathon. Fast forward a year or so and I have been forced to eat those words.

I'm still not sure what came over me, but I decided to Google ultra-races soon after crossing the finish line at the London Marathon in April 2017. I blame post-marathon delirium, combined with a large dose of intrigue and a dollop of naivety. I thought that if I was (hypothetically, obviously) ever going to do an ultra-marathon I wanted the race to be: a) relatively soon, so as to capitalise on the fitness I had banked for the London Marathon; b) close to my home town of Bristol so as not to inconvenience my family and reduce any logistical headaches; and c) definitely less than 62 miles. Scheduled for mid-June, taking place along the Cotswold Way and a (meagre, according to Vassos) 52-miles, the 'Race to the Tower' ticked all the boxes.

I entered. And then became concerned. The longest run I'd ever done was a marathon and, off-road, I'd completed the 22-mile Man Versus Horse a few years ago. Runners racing against riders on horseback in Wales. I didn't beat the horse, but I had thoroughly enjoyed pitting myself against the equines across the Welsh hills. But 52 miles was an altogether different kettle of fish. Could I finish it? Was I strong enough? What would I eat? What should I wear? What on earth was I thinking? Will Vassos lend me his running rucksack? So, yes, doing an ultra definitely scared me. But this was part of its appeal. I like to be pushed out of my comfort zone and do things I think I might not be able to do. It's an important message to send my daughter and to others. We may not be confident in our ability to succeed, but this shouldn't stop us trying.

A double marathon completed, I can now reflect on my virgin ultra experience. I loved the rawness of the event, I felt unburdened (unlike triathlon) with kit or gadgets and really appreciated the informal, relaxed atmosphere. I realised that, whilst ultras had seemed impossible or inconceivable, they are truly open to all, with people of all backgrounds and abilities taking part – from the speedsters at the pointy end to those out for a rather long walk closer to the back. The camaraderie between everyone was fantastic, and it was the least intimidating race environment I think I have ever encountered.

I also really liked not running to a target pace, and focusing more on the journey than on specific times/splits/positions, etc. Of course, I tried my hardest but I really couldn't have specific time or outcome goals, other than to finish, which was very liberating. In terms of race strategy, I slowed down, walked up the steep hills, fuelled early on and learnt how to smell the flowers, look around me and enjoy the entire experience, rather than only the destination.

And yes, a month later I did my second ultra, the off-road, hilly 30-mile Mendip Marauder, from Wells to Weston-super-Mare in Somerset, which was a wonderful, low-key, local (for me) race. It took in many of the places I know well, having done a lot of cycling around those hills. We travelled along paths paved with stinging nettles, through dense forests and over boggy grasslands. We climbed for views over the Welsh Estuary and descended to the beach at Uphill where the ubiquitous Mr Whippy awaited. Being a relatively short 30 miles, it also meant I finished in time to head back to a friend's BBQ, and refuel with a burger and a glass of wine before the sun had started to go down.

I know there will be many more ultras in my future, as much for the journey as the destination.

– Chrissie Wellington

start line

I was told the following tale by my grandfather, as I sat on his knee one sweltering summer afternoon in the house he built by the sea. For a long time I believed it was Ancient Greek wisdom, passed down from generation to generation. I liked to think you could trace its origins back through the mists of our family, through Cretan mountains and remote island fishing ports, way back through time to the great Athenian empire, to the dawn of philosophy and civilisation. Back in fact, to the original ultra-runners. To those legendary long distance messengers like Pheidippides, the greatest of them all and the inspiration for what we now call the Marathon.

But as it turns out, it's actually a famous Cherokee parable from Tennessee.

> An old man is teaching his grandson about life. 'A fight is going on inside me,' he explains to the boy. 'It is a terrible fight and it is between two wolves. One is evil – he is anger, envy, sorrow, regret, arrogance, self-pity, resentment and ego. The other is good – he is joy, peace, love, hope, determination, humility, fortitude, compassion and truth.
>
> 'The same fight is going on inside you – and inside every other person, too.'
>
> The boy thinks about it for a minute and then asks his grandfather, 'Which wolf will win?'
>
> The old Cherokee smiles and replies simply: 'The one you feed.'

And that's the point of this really. All this endless running. All the wonderful people who enter all these stupidly long races knowing they'll frequently fail to finish. All the pain they suffer, all the injuries, the failures. All the lost toenails.

And also the successes. The feeling of having pushed yourself to the edge of your limitations – and deciding not to quit. To push on regardless. To keep on running. The satisfaction of helping a fellow runner in trouble; the comfort of being helped. The lifelong friendships formed. The exhilaration of getting your body to achieve the impossible. You break yourself down, like stripping an engine, yet somehow emerge more whole.

I don't much like the term 'ultra-running' because it sounds exclusive, which is the opposite of what it should be, and is. Endurance running is inclusive and quietly seems to make you a better version of yourself. For me and so many of the runners I've spoken to over the years, running long gives a powerful sense of joy and serenity.

There's the warm blanket of community too. The generosity and positivity of runners and volunteers, as well as supportive, long-suffering friends and family behind the scenes. On the trail, there's the slow accumulation of problems, and even slower process of solving them, little by little, one by one. You're absolutely in the moment. It can be like therapy, or an exorcism. A journey of self-knowledge. You're feeling liberated from daily life but you're also taking control, escaping into a more simple world. After all, we were born to run.

I'm a father to three terrific children. When each of them came into the world (respectively in March 2004, May 2006 and June 2014), I experienced a deep sense of contentment that stuck around for weeks. It seemed like everything was going to be OK and nothing could burst my private bubble of joy.

When I completed my first 100-mile race, I felt that same elation crossing the finishing line. Even as I mildly convulsed in the car on the way home (I wasn't driving, thankfully) I had a great big grin on my face. For a month or more, I was telling everyone who'd listen how amazing it is to run a hundred miles in one go. How they should try it.

And so they should. I know it sounds like a long way and of course it is. If you'd told me five years ago that I'd be running these silly distances, I simply wouldn't have believed you. But it comes in stages. First-ever run, then first 5K, 10K, half-marathon, marathon... and anything beyond 26.2 miles is an ultra. Just build it up slowly. You don't have to be a full-time athlete to run a hundred miles. After all, it's only running. And running. And not stopping. How hard can it be?

Reaching the finishing line is exquisite. Life-affirming and renewing. But the journey can be so very tough, and the urge to stop overwhelming. So why do we put ourselves through it? Simple really. We're feeding the good wolf.

1. athens

Athens, early evening, and there's a minor commotion at the pre-race briefing. Several hundred crack ultra-runners are assembled in a slightly too small hotel conference room. They're going to attempt to run 153 miles the following morning. And they're worried about breakfast.

A toned, capable-looking Swede sitting next to me raises a lean, tanned arm.

'You want us to get on the buses at 5:45am, yes?'

The race director rolls his eyes and nods. He looks exactly like the bride's father in *My Big Fat Greek Wedding*. Sounds the same too, with a Greek accent straight from central casting. He tries unsuccessfully to stop himself sounding patronising and sighs as he replies.

'Once again, you need to be at the start at the Acropolis at 6 o'clock. It is 15 minutes away on the bus, so please – be on the bus at 5:45. Please! It is not... *what is the word*... difficult.'

The Swede, I sense, has the backing of the entire room when he replies. This is important stuff. Don't get between an ultra-runner and their breakfast on the day of a big race.

'But I've checked with the hotel, which is the official race hotel where you've organised for us to stay, and they won't open breakfast until 5:45. So please, what do you suggest we should do?'

The director looks momentarily nonplussed. A pause, then a mischievous twinkle appears in the corners of his eyes.

'Well, what I suggest is...' A Mediterranean shrug now, and a smile. 'Eat quickly.'

I suspect I'm one of few runners in the room who finds this funny. My snort of laughter attracts several derisive glances. Like I say, never get between an ultra-runner and their race-day breakfast.

I further suspect that the race itself, all 36 hours of it, will prove to be a bit like the race director's breakfast solution – amusingly haphazard, charming, ever so slightly chaotic... basically, very Greek. And I say that as a Greek.

On that score, I'll be proved utterly wrong. Everything works like a dream. The volunteers are the most joyful, helpful and efficient I've ever encountered. The atmosphere from Athens to Corinth to Nemea to Sparta, through villages, past schools, over a mountain, is exhilarating; is immense. Throughout the 153 miles, 75 aid stations, police cordons, road signs, mountain rescue, doctors, physios, photographers... the whole race, a logistical nightmare, runs like clockwork. I do too, for some of it.

But for the moment, on the eve of the 35th Spartathlon, there's the breakfast situation to add to the significant list of worries already churning my every thought. Principal among these is, how on earth do I, a relative newbie, expect to complete what many consider to be the world's toughest running race? Only around a third finish, and everybody who starts is a serious ultra-runner with a proven pedigree. There are strict qualifying criteria to get into the race, which I have satisfied, but only just.

The briefing ends and I return to the small Athenian bedroom I'm sharing with a friendly Aussie called Mick. He has an old-fashioned RAF-style moustache and boasts a top-three finish in the one of the few other races with a realistic claim on the title 'world's toughest', the Badwater 135.* Mick's prepared methodically for this. Meanwhile I very much fear I'm about to be found out.

---

* Badwater is a 135-mile single-stage race held in California's Death Valley every July, when temperatures can reach 50 degrees (120°F). It begins some 300 feet below sea level and ends 8,000 feet higher, near the top of Mount Whitney. Each runner must be accompanied throughout by a crew of at least two people and a van. According to Badwater lore, the roads are sometimes so hot that you have to run on the white line in the middle to stop the soles of your shoes melting. It's a battle against heat, rather than time, with a generous 48-hour limit.

The Spartathlon doesn't take prisoners. It's not just the inexperienced or under-prepared who fail here; they're not even on the start line. This is *Top Gun* for distance runners. But even the best of the best come a cropper on the unforgiving road from Athens to Sparta, and a list of those who've floundered between the two historic cities reads like a who's who of ultra-running. Badwater has frightening heat, but it's a combination of factors that makes the Spartathlon so brutal. First there's the prodigious length – an awful lot can go wrong in 153 miles. Then there's the 4,000-foot mountain, which has to be climbed and descended at night. The weather can be gruesome – often swelteringly hot, frequently very wet – sometimes both in the same race. And most of all, it's the cut-offs – 75 checkpoints, one every two miles, and each must be reached within a strict time limit. If you're late, they simply ask you to hand in your number and that's where your race ends. To make matters worse, those cut-offs make you push hard early on (just over four hours to complete the first marathon, just over nine for the first 50 miles), which can be fatal to your chances later on. It's a race designed to mess with your head as well as your legs. A baffling, unfathomable, elongated, enigmatic athletic conundrum.

It also has history. This is no arbitrary run between two random places. In fact in many ways, the Spartathlon is The Race.

Most people know the story about the unfortunate Ancient Greek messenger, Pheidippides, who ran all the way from Marathon to Athens, 26-odd miles, and died as soon as he arrived. He was carrying news of a significant military victory and that journey, of course, gave birth to what we now call the Marathon. Two and a half thousand years after his death, millions take on the 26.2-mile challenge every year, and Pheidippides' legacy is complete.

Only, he's a little derided isn't he? Poor old Pheidippides – the professional messenger who couldn't survive a gentle jog from Marathon to Athens...

A few days earlier, the Athenians had become aware of a massive Persian army coming ashore at Marathon. The Persians, brutal and bloodthirsty, had been conquering all before them. Only Athens and Sparta hadn't yet fallen or surrendered. On hearing of the impending invasion, Athens would have been in the grip of a widespread panic. A Persian victory wouldn't just mean an end to democracy and civilisation, both still relatively new concepts. On a personal level, it would have been terrifying. All the men – fathers, husbands, sons – would be killed or castrated. Women and children faced rape and enslavement. The Persians, there were just so many of them. They seemed invincible.

The only thing for it was to ask Sparta, a rival city state, for help. Together perhaps they had a glimmer of hope. Time was critical, but of course this was 500BC – there would be no phoning for help, no SOS text or tweeting @Sparta. The only way to get word 150 miles over the mountains to the Peloponnese was to send a messenger, a runner. Pheidippides was the best they had. With the hopes of a nation and the future of democracy riding on his shoulders, as well as the safety of his family, he set off from Athens. According to Herodotus, the great historian of Ancient Greece, Pheidippides arrived in Sparta 'before night fell on the second day'.

That was the start of his epic run. His return home from Marathon a few days later was the end. There was a middle bit too, and we'll get to that.

But fast forward several thousand years, to a young RAF officer called John Foden reading Herodotus whilst on leave in Greece. 'By Jove!' he thinks. 'Running such a distance in a day and a half… is that even possible?' This was 1982, and Foden decided to give it a shot. He reached Sparta in a remarkable 37 hours, 37 minutes, his exploits captured the imagination of the locals, and the Spartathlon was born.

So on the eve of the 35th edition, we're preparing to recreate Pheidippides' epic journey that had much to do with preserving freedom, democracy and civilisation. That objective, those principles, still resonate today. Especially today. But I do wish my roommate would stop farting.

Mick's blowing wind approximately once every three minutes, which is significantly more than ideal in a cramped hotel room. He has a stomach upset and says he can't help it. Mick is the only Australian in the field this year, and I'm officially part of the Greek contingent. I was told my chances of getting through the entry ballot would be greater if I brandished my Greek passport rather than my British one (not true as it turns out, but I got lucky). The GB team are all staying together in a neighbouring hotel and the Greek runners don't seem to need one. So Mick and I have been thrown together and having spent the past 24 hours in each other's company, eating meals, going shopping, we've basically – despite the unfortunate smell in here – become firm friends.

Mick looks bewildered as I hold up two pairs of shorts and ask him which he thinks I should run in tomorrow: the posh new ones, or the trusty old ones. He can't understand why I wouldn't have worked this out weeks ago. Indeed why I'd even contemplate wearing new shorts for a race like this. Mick and I have almost the opposite approach to pre-race preparation. He'll plot, plan and science his way to the start line; I'll wing it. He has a nutrition plan for the race; I'll eat and drink whatever's available. And he's got a folder with laminated sheets detailing the exact location of each of the 75 aid stations, including which side of the street he needs to be running on, what the cut-off times are and what provisions they're likely to stock; I'll just see how I go.

But I fear my 'wing it' strategy, which has served me well in races all the way up to 100 miles, is about to be exposed. Especially as I don't have anyone with me. Most other runners have a crew in a hire car to meet and help them at 17 pre-approved points along the route. I'm feeling under-prepared and alone. But I know how pernicious negative thoughts can be, so I try to remind myself about the positives. As far as I can tell, this is a race that might suit me. I know I have the speed; a sub-three-hour marathon is almost a pre-requisite here. I know I have the mental toughness. And I know I probably have the endurance too. I've done all the training I physically had time for: I've run my commutes; I've completed a hilly 50-mile race and felt I could run on beyond the

5

finish (which I didn't, I went for fish and chips instead); I sacrificed siestas in France to go on long, hot, hilly, holiday runs; and just three weeks ago I had a few hours to myself and simply kept running around and around London's tiny Holland Park until I'd racked up 35 miles.

Then again, few people finish Spartathlon, especially on their first attempt. I keep vacillating wildly between cautious confidence and utter terror. For some reason I know a DNF (Did Not Finish) will really sting here. The hours to the start tick by ever so slowly.

A night filled with a nervous lack of sleep (and many farts) later, and it's time to get up. My breakfast strategy is to attempt to charm my way – in Greek – into the hotel buffet before it officially opens. It works, and I fill my boots. One last-minute change of mind about which shorts to wear later (I sensibly opt for the tried and tested) and I'm in a good mood as we line up in the darkness outside the hotel to board the bus to the Acropolis. I've never been more desperate for a race to be under way.

They say the Spartathlon doesn't really begin until halfway, so not until after night falls again this evening, but at least when we start running in an hour or so, I'll be able to answer several burning questions. I'll know for instance how my legs will feel when they're in motion. I'll know whether I've got any niggles and how badly they're likely to affect me. And most of all, I'll be able to put all this nervous energy to good use. This has been my longest-ever taper: I've run just once in six days, and not at all for four. When I did last run – what was meant to be a gentle jog round my usual four-mile home loop – I accidentally took almost a minute off my course record. I'm fit to burst.

The start of the Spartathlon is truly colossal. I never thought you could beat the way we once set off on a trail half-marathon in Keswick – taking a highly polished, beautiful wooden boat across the dark, calm waters of Derwentwater in the Lake District for a dawn departure on a distant shore. But this is different gravy.

As the sun comes up over Athens, 400 eager runners stand in the chill shadow of the greatest enduring symbol of Ancient Greece – a tribute to democracy, freedom and civilisation. We're about to embark on as near as possible an exact recreation of a run 2,500 years ago whose purpose was to save those ideals. The finger of history seems to be pointing expectantly at each and every one of us. Perhaps that's why the atmosphere is so charged. Time seems to stall. I check my watch – 25 minutes to go. Ten minutes later I check again – 24 minutes to go. It's almost unbearable.

Runners say final farewells to their support teams, a drone hovers overhead taking photos, camera crews mill amongst us filming everything. They've come from all corners of the earth to run this race and despite the obvious language barriers, there's tremendous camaraderie and plenty of random hugging. I'm a big fan of random hugging and enter the fray with gusto. Finally, *finally*, as the 10-second countdown begins, two Japanese men to my right are so overwrought, they let out primal roars. Others join in. The 2017 Spartathlon begins to the soundtrack of a battlefield.

The joy of being in motion courses through my legs. The only advice I've heard over and over in the days and weeks leading up to this is: *don't set off too quickly*. I set off far too quickly. I can't help it. It's the release of pent-up energy and emotion, plus the glory of these early miles. I know Athens well, but I've never met *this* Athens. There are police stopping traffic at every junction and the local commuters, not widely known for their patience, happily wait behind cordons, lean out of car windows and shout '*Bravo!*' as runners go by. The honks we get are supportive, not aggressive. People at bus stops, in shops and tavernas, they all smile, encourage and applaud. Outside of Greece, only the ultra-running community really knows about the Spartathlon. Here everybody's heard of it. Greeks are proud of this race, and feel strongly that you're honouring their culture and history simply by participating. Which of course we are.

Athens is twice the size of London in terms of area. It disappears in a flash. Suddenly we're running through countryside and entering a large village. School's out for Sparta. Kids are lining the street offering high-fives and loud cheers of encouragement. When I reply in Greek

('*Opa!*' I shout, it's an expression of simple joy), the roars double in volume. This is just great. I speed up. I can't help it – it's like the support is aimed directly at my leg muscles. Every '*Bravo!*', every '*Kalo dromo*' (safe journey) and every '*Kali epitixia*' (good luck) seems to increase my pace ever so slightly. Past full marathon distance in three and a half hours; I fear this is unsustainably quick.

We reach the coast, heavy industry country, and we're running on the main road amongst the lorries. On a usual Friday morning this would be suicidal, but the drivers mostly seem to be expecting us and generally give Spartathletes a wide berth, usually accompanied by a honk of good luck.

The imposing refineries give way to a glorious pebbly bay. The green-blue waters, a strong wind rippling the surface, are begging to be swum in. To add to the allure, the next village is called Neraki – which means 'a little bit of water'. Whilst running, about 30 miles in, I chat to my good friend and colleague Chris Evans on the Radio 2 Breakfast Show. He asks one question, *How's it going?* – my enthusiastic, endorphin-fuelled reply goes on for several minutes.

Still cars and lorries hoot their support and pedestrians shout '*Bravo!*' Another school gives kids the morning off lessons to cheer for the runners and offer high-fives. Dozens of them set up camp under a road bridge for maximum volume: these '*Opa*'s have echoes. Again, I can't help but run still quicker. I hope I don't end up paying for this pace later in the race. Although I suspect (correctly) that I will.

Scott Jurek also worried about how fast he was going as he won the Spartathlon three times in a row. When I catch up with him one midweek morning, he's at home at the foot of the Rocky Mountains of Colorado with his happy, noisy, young daughter. I'd heard he was a nice guy, and he proves it immediately. He's profusely, genuinely apologetic about being just a few minutes late.

When we start chatting about the Spartathlon, his enthusiasm is self-evident. After all it takes a special sort of race to persuade someone of Scott's calibre to make a 12,000-mile round trip three years running.

For me it was trying to obviously get a better performance each time, or run a little faster, kind of gauge how I stacked up against somebody like the great Yiannis Kouros*. Having that opportunity to run against legends on the same course, and in that environment.

Even though I'm more of a trail mountain guy, I think the Spartathlon is a special event with the people, the culture – it really celebrates all of those aspects. Yes, there was a race I tried to win and to do better each year, but there's a surreal sense of culture and history there that is unique. A lot of ultras in the US are pretty old, in one sense of old – but something like the Spartathlon, it revels in that history and depth.

And the people... Greece is known for their long distance runners, and the community and the people really celebrate all the athletes as if they are Olympians. The Olympic spirit is still alive there. So that's what's super special about going to the Spartathlon. And you know, winning three times is great, but experiencing the culture each time was to me, I think, the real prize.

Scott pinpoints two especially memorable experiences on the long road to Sparta. The first was 115 miles into the 2007 race when he put in a burst to overtake a Polish adversary who'd been leading since the start. Scott was running unsustainably fast, but knew how demoralising it can be when you're passed by someone moving at a pace you can't match. He's a truly nice guy, Scott Jurek, but an equally fierce competitor – he'll always take an opportunity to demoralise an opponent. Scott opened up a big lead and assumed the race was won.

---

* Yiannis Kouros, or the 'Running God', is a Greek ultra-runner who holds numerous records from 100 to 1,000 miles and from 12 hours to six days. A multiple Spartathlon champion, he says his secret is cast-iron mental strength. 'I take over my body with my mind. I tell it that it's not tired and it listens.' He holds the record for the three fastest Spartathlon times; Scott Jurek's three wins put him fourth, fifth and sixth on the all-time list. When Kouros won his first Spartathlon in 1984, nobody believed his record. It was simply too fast – humanly impossible. So he came back the following year and ran faster.

So it came as a shock, several 7-minute miles later, to see another runner's headlamp a hundred yards behind him and closing fast. He put the hammer down, risked everything to run flat out. But the Pole was nothing if not resilient, he simply refused to be shaken off. Eight maxed-out miles later, Scott realised the truth – that the torchlight behind him didn't belong to the Pole, or any other Spartathlete come to that, but a bandit runner who'd jumped onto the course with a marathon to go. Scott was understandably a little upset (and a lot exhausted) but still hung on to win.

I think it's a great example of separating negative thoughts from reality. Thinking 'I can't do this, I can't go on, I can't push a little harder'. But you still have another gear. And that to me sums up the atmosphere of the Spartathlon. It really squeezes the best out of everyone. And ultra-events in general force you to find that extra bit of energy that you didn't think you had.

And one other story. I was running alone through this small, tiny village, maybe 10, 15 houses, and a woman came running out to me, asking me if I wanted 'pagos, nero' [ice, water]. It was blistering hot, the heat of the afternoon, and I remember her coming out with ice cold water and then she also brought some basil.

She started putting the basil in my hair and rubbing it on my arms. I've never experienced anything like it. Basil has healing properties. It really made me think of Hippocrates and the Greek traditions. Also the Mediterranean cuisine and the deep knowledge of certain herbs and plants. I couldn't understand what she was saying but I knew she was trying to expose some healing energy with the power of the herb. To me, as somebody who loves food, loves the cultural aspects, it was really a neat way of experiencing that first-hand.

In fact Scott's love of food, vegan food, is legendary. You only need to read the title of his terrific first book to get the idea: *Eat & Run*. Every chapter ends with one of his recipes. My own favourite is the Chocolate Adzuki Bar.

He wasn't the most obvious candidate to turn to a vegan (he prefers the term plant-based) diet. He was given a rifle by his father and soon knew how to shoot, kill, skin, gut and cook an animal. As a kid, with the exception of tinned sweetcorn, he hated all vegetables. But early in his running career, Scott realised that the food he was eating had a massive impact on his athletic performance, and that cutting out animal products from his diet basically helped turn him into a winner.

Some 15 years after he turned vegan, he's delighted to see more and more people finally following his lead.

Yeah, it's more acceptable. You're not considered weird and laughed at. I mean I was like a hippie, most people would say. But it's not just for health nuts and hippies. I think because it's become more mainstream and people look differently at food in general, to maybe 20 years ago.

It's really encouraging to see that people are looking at lifestyle and health and wellness as a whole. These things go hand in hand with running. We see people who come to the sport who weren't runners, who didn't have a reason *per se* to run, but they picked it up. So I think it's a really exciting time, not only for diet, but also for wellness and lifestyle. There's hope for us humans to perhaps solve some of these preventable diseases.

This is something I'm keen to explore with Scott. It seems his holistic view of food has echoes in his outlook to his chosen sport. I ask him what he loves most about running such long distances.

I get a very simplified way of living and kind of get to go back in time, where I'm moving my body and becoming more animal-like. It's really about being unplugged in this modern day and age. Although technology is great – I even occasionally listen to music – I love just being able to tap into the sounds and sights around me. Doing long-distance events or just training and running in the woods and on the trails – it's basically knowing that I'm not going to be in control. Having to surrender to the elements.

11

And there are skills and things that we're losing because we're always comfortable. We like to be in control as humans. In modern day society we live in a very controlled environment where we have heating systems, and air conditioning, and we have cars…. We don't have to use our bodies. When I'm running I feel like I'm keeping that intuition and adaptability at the forefront of my existence. Being uncomfortable, I believe, is a benefit.

This is fun. This is hard work. This is joy. My first ultra-marathon was a 50 miler. It was a new thing, a new way to explore. And there is that element of exploration. Not certain if I could do something.

And then I enjoyed the winning, too. Seeing what my body could do. Could I push it further? I knew that this was good for me, that I was getting something out of it. At first I don't think I had that same appreciation, but I learned more throughout the years and became more attuned to the other benefits.

My hope is that the sport continues to grow. But I hope with that growth and with that discovery, we don't see a loss of history and tradition. It feels sometimes like some people think, 'if it didn't happen in the age of the Internet, or we don't have video of it, then it didn't happen'.

I started the sport when there was only one monthly publication. The Internet was still in its infancy. I would hope that the traditions and the real heart of the sport continue to flourish. This is more than certain events, or winning, or what's hot, or who has more followers on social media.

The sport didn't happen in the last 15 years. People often think this is a new sport. I look to a lot of the great heroes of the past. There are a lot of ultra-runners, even in the UK, who don't even know who Don Ritchie* is. And Don was one of the legends – and still is to this day.

---

* Don Ritchie is one of endurance running's great pioneers. Born in Scotland in 1944, he's held no fewer than 14 world records including 50km, 50 miles, 100km, 100 miles, 200km and 24 Hours Indoor. Voted the finest ultra-runner of the 20th century, he was still competitive in his fifties, frequently racing against people 30 years his junior.

My hope is that in future we continue to grow but still retain that history and we remember the legends of the sport. It's really about a culture and a people. I have great hope and faith that it won't change. Races are harder to get into, we have lotteries now to get into a lot of the popular races. But the sport at its core is the same.

And nowhere does the sport honour its traditions more than it does here, on the streets of Greece. On the long climb towards Corinth, an elderly man holds up a sign at a road junction. It's in English: *'Thank you Spartathletes for honouring our country'*. Wow.

I check my watch as soon afterwards I find myself running over a vertiginous yellow footbridge. I'm crossing the Corinth Canal and it's a magnificent sight. Vertical rock sides rise 300 feet from the sea. The canal saves the 450-mile trip around the Peloponnese, but it's too narrow for modern ocean freighters so most of its traffic is now tourist ships. No sign of any now though, nor of the clever submersible bridge which apparently opens underwater. Just my watch beeping to tick off another mile and warn me that I'm massively ahead of schedule.

Don't bank time, they told me, the experienced runners and especially those who'd failed to finish this before. *In the first third of the race, don't get to the cut-offs too early or you'll pay for it later.* It's common knowledge that the initial cut-offs are brutal, so the trick is to use all of the nine-and-a-bit hours you're allowed for the first 50 miles. Well, Corinth signals the end of the first third of the race, 50 miles down, just over 100 to go. Perhaps not even the end of the beginning in running terms – but a milestone nonetheless. Ideally I'd have liked to arrive here in around eight and a half hours. My watch says seven.

I'm going way too fast.

2. botolphs

I'm 61 miles into a 100-mile running race across the beautiful South Downs of England. It's late on Saturday afternoon, some 10 hours since the start of the race, and my biggest problem is a blister forming below a toenail. It's urgent and has to be sorted like, now!

This has happened to me before. It's a little painful when you're running on it, and a little more painful when you're not. For a few days it will look properly disgusting as it starts to peel away from under the skin. Kids will squirm delightedly as you show them the nail flapping around, loosely connected to the foot only at the very top corner of the toe. If you stub the toe or anyone steps on it, it hurts like the end of the world. Eventually, after a week or two, and probably as you pull on your socks in the morning, the nail will come off completely and that'll be that.

In the world of ultra-running, it's a tiny pinprick of a problem. Barely worth mentioning. But like I say, it's apparently crucial that I deal with it immediately. And to make matters worse, it's not even my own toe.

I'm not running, you see, not today. I ran this last year – my debut over 100 miles and I loved every second of the 19-plus hours it took me to haul myself along the famously pretty path through the chalk hills from Winchester to Eastbourne. Today I'm back at the South Downs Way 100 (SDW100) volunteering. Helping run Aid Station Eight, or Botolphs as we're officially known.

There are six of us helping out here. Five normal human beings and a force of nature called Sarah. She greets every runner, every single one of the tired, dirty, bedraggled, sometimes grumpy, often bloody, always sweaty competitors, she greets them all with a loud cheer and a hug. Somehow as they approach, she speedily looks up their names from her list of race numbers and makes each of them feel like their arrival has made her day.

The ones she knows personally, and there are loads of these, they get a cheer and a banshee shriek as if their presence, at that moment in that place, has realised all of Sarah's lifelong dreams and ambitions. Difficult to imagine a better way to reach an aid station really. Now we've met and she knows me, I'm determined to run the next race she volunteers at, just for her happy hug and to hear my name being whooped, shrieked and squealed. People like Sarah (and her husband Tom who also volunteers but less loudly) are the lifeblood of this fast-growing sport. It's a privilege to be volunteering with them for the first time.

Mind you, it's not easy. Not when you've been on your feet for 12 hours and someone wants you to pop a blister under her toenail.

'You do know I'm not a doctor?'

'Yep!'

'And you know that none of us here has any medical training whatsoever, that we're all just runners helping out for the day? Oh, and we also have zero medical equipment.'

'Yes. But you've got a needle because I can see a safety pin on the table over there. So please would you sort out the blister?'

'You're absolutely sure about this?'

'I am absolutely sure.'

'Totally and completely convinced?'

'Yes, totally and completely convinced.'

Though thankfully, in the end, she isn't. She sits down on one of our fold-up chairs, whips off her left shoe and changes her mind (hooray!) as she begins removing her sock. Possibly the idea of having to put the foul-smelling sock back on again makes her think better of it. Or perhaps it's watching my rudimentary attempt at needle sterilisation in warm water from the teapot.

Either way, she accepts some sandwiches and sweets from our lavish selection and listens sceptically as I explain that the same thing happened to me a few weeks back in the mountains of Wales, and what's likely to happen to her toe and nail. I try to cheer her up by promising the toe's unlikely to be her biggest problem in the 39 miles she has left to run, but I'm not sure how much that helps. She looks decidedly forlorn as she sets off up the hill towards the next aid station. I sincerely hope for her sake that by the time she gets there, she'll have had a little win. Or at the very least, that the volunteers prove generally less incompetent and more encouraging than I've just been.

The aid stations are absolutely key. In a race as long as 100 miles, you have to break it down into chunks or it can seem overwhelming. So you're running from checkpoint to checkpoint, aid station to aid station, and every time you reach one it's a significant victory. Whenever you depart, full of fruit, crisps and flat cola, you're embarking on another adventure.

Mile 61 is a good place to be – far enough into the race for runners to be beginning to struggle and suitably grateful for your presence, but far enough from the finish that the end is still vague, abstract, hypothetical.

We arrived here at lunchtime, us volunteers, though I was a bit late and missed the delivery of equipment. I'm never late, not since I once missed kick-off in a football match I was covering for student radio. But I'd just been camping with my son and dramatically underestimated the time it takes to round up eight 11-year-old boys playing in the woods by a river. So when I finally reached Botolphs, I was greeted by five people huddled around a huge wire container recently regurgitated from a large white lorry. Inside, haphazardly arranged, a gazebo, two fold-up tables, six enormous water containers, a gas stove, kettle, tea urn, some flags, route markers and a huge box of general supplies (gaffer tape, kitchen roll, plastic ties, paper plates, salt tablets and lots of isotonic powder ready for mixing).

As for the food, masses and masses and masses of it, we've brought it all ourselves: white bread (eight loaves), two tubs of butter, dozens of tortilla wraps, jam, peanut butter, sausage rolls, scotch eggs, cheese, biscuits, chocolate, crisps, sweets, fruit, nuts, more crisps, more sweets, and gallons and gallons of Coke. No wonder they say ultras are like children's parties. Crisps, sweets, squash and cola – and lots of running around.

First things first, find somewhere to set up. Easier said than done on a sunny Saturday afternoon – free parking and the splendour of the South Downs stretching for miles in either direction combine to make our lay-by unusually packed with parked cars. The only free space is at the far end, outside a grand country house a quarter of a mile in the opposite direction from the race route. This poses a problem: put the aid station too far off track, and runners will understandably grumble about the added yardage. So for a short time we simply stand idly around, staring at a long line of parked cars and willing their owners to return and move them.

Almost at once, a blue Volvo estate and an old-style yellow Mini are reunited with their drivers who leave us the perfect double space to set up shop.

I say perfect. I mean almost perfect. On the plus side, it's precisely positioned where the South Downs Way joins the lay-by. The only issue being the enormous thorn bush which will need to house half of the gazebo if we aren't going to block the road. Someone will need to get very well acquainted with the brambles. Somehow, almost imperceptibly and I'm still wondering how it happened, I'm selected as thorn bush correspondent.

Try as I might, I can't overturn this decision. Thorns and me have previous. I was once surprised whilst running the marathon section of an Ironman triathlon by a sudden, desperate and urgent need to relieve myself. And I'm afraid we're talking number twos here. I had literally seconds to choose where to go. In a blind panic, I took stock of my immediate surroundings: the urge had struck as I ran along a busy towpath next to some children playing on a green. I realised to my horror that the only real option was the large, deep thorn bush between the path and the River Trent. On that occasion, having dived like Tom Daley into the spikes, I emerged bloody and in pain – but thrilled not to have disgraced myself in public. This time, I had both

17

longer to think about it and less personal motivation to get involved in the sharp stuff.

However, my fellow volunteers – all otherwise nice people – decided that I was absolutely the man for this unwelcome task. Perhaps because I'd arrived late: last in, first in the bush. So whilst they grin benignly, I gingerly step into the vicious shrub carrying two fully extended legs of our enormous gazebo. Fair to say that when I emerge several sweary minutes later, I look like I've done battle with a particularly vicious kitten. But the whole episode (and I admit I milked it for extra effect) does seem to unite us – listening to a grown man cursing and yelping will do that to a group.

We have several hours to get ready for the arrival of the runners and prepare the food as if Heston himself is looking over our shoulders. Never has strawberry jam been spread as carefully over peanut butter on flatbread. (If you've never tried a jam and peanut butter wrap by the way, and I know it doesn't sound or indeed look particularly appealing, then you're missing out big time.) Fruits are surgically peeled and sliced. And we even cut up the five green peppers left over from my camping trip the night before – I'd optimistically brought them along in the hope the boys might eat some veg with their sausages; they were predictably ignored.

The first runner to reach us is in a tearing hurry. He's heard his lead over his nearest challenger is disappearing mile by mile, so he hops impatiently from foot to foot as he waits for us to replenish his water bottles. As soon as we have, he tears off up the hill, stuffing them into his running vest as he goes. Runner number two is far more laid back, smiling, strong, radiating confidence. The difference between hunter and hunted. He spends a little longer with us and exchanges a few pleasantries before setting off. The lead changes hands somewhere on the undulating, chalky road to Aid Station Nine.

Back at Eight, nobody touches our lovingly prepared food for an hour or more. We're just beginning to take it personally when the 'competers' are replaced with the far more numerous 'completers'. From a volunteer's point of view, this is more like it. We suddenly get busy. And I do mean busy.

No longer are there four of us hanging around while one or two fill bottles with water and/or sport drink. Now the runners arrive in droves and it takes all six of us operating on full power to cope. Everyone wants their fluid bottles topping up. Some want crisps, others sweets, watermelon or cheese. The peanut butter and jam wraps prove particularly popular. Several runners ask for salt tablets or cola. Most have smiles on their faces and a deeply determined look in their eyes. A few announce their race is run and can't be persuaded to carry on. There's the woman who wants a blister popping before changing her mind. A man strips to his waist and produces a clean, dry running shirt from his backpack, binning his old one. Another fellow gets confused between water and cola and accidentally cools off by dousing himself in sticky brown liquid. A few kind souls, who've heard on the radio about the damage I've done to my ankle during a recent multi-stage mountain ultra, enquire about how it's healing. Food supplies become decimated. The watermelon is the first to run out, closely followed by the wraps. Sandwich supplies are low, mini scotch eggs are cut in half then quarters to make them last longer, and only the pumpkin seeds are left from the once overflowing dried fruit, nut and seed bowl. And still, everybody ignores the green peppers.

We volunteers encourage, cajole, applaud and cheer the runners on their way. As it begins to get dark, the stove comes into its own. Those arriving now have little chance of earning the coveted *100 Miles – One Day* belt buckle for finishing in under 24 hours. They're aiming for the *100 Miles – Finisher* buckle and thus have time to sit down for a cup of sweet tea. When you've run 61 miles, it's astonishing how sweet you'll want your tea. I think an early request of five sugars can't be beaten, until someone asks me to prepare them a small cup with seven.

After a long while, we're back down to a trickle of runners. Two volunteers depart, one for home, the other to help at the finishing line. The Downs are now pitch dark. We can see the runners approach from a mile away via the slowly moving dots of light from their head torches. Sarah is constantly on the phone to earlier aid stations and carefully notes which runners have abandoned elsewhere so we know how many we're still expecting. As midnight approaches, we've got just three left to come in.

Two men arrive looking utterly bedraggled and sit down for a long time drinking tea, eating what's left of our food and turning their backs on the green peppers. They're still well inside the official cut-off time but don't look like they have another 39 miles left in their ailing legs. We're in two minds whether to encourage them to continue, but you never know, they might get a second wind. I walk with them to the foot of the next hill and wish them well. For the first time all day, I don't wish I was running too. Marshalling has been hard enough.

Pretty much all organised sport wouldn't happen without volunteers, but that's especially true of ultra-running. The company that organises the SDW100, Centurion, puts on eight races a year – four 100-milers and four 50s. They need up to 140 volunteers for every single race to make them work. The people who give up their time to help are often injured runners investing their energies in a positive way, those hoping for a discount off a future entry fee, or people like me who want to give something back having relied on volunteers in the past.

Same story at parkrun. The hugely popular and absolutely phenomenal free, weekly, timed 5km race in a park near you simply would not happen without volunteers. Of course it's brilliant that someone chooses to give up his or her time to help other people achieve their sporting goals. But what's in it for them?

Chantel Scherer is one of the world's top experts on volunteering. I catch up with her a few minutes after she's been to a big meeting about how to deliver a successful Olympic Games, and about an hour before she's due to go on holiday. Chantel helps run Join In, which is the national brand for local sports volunteering. She's one of those people who truly loves and believes in what they're doing, and her enthusiasm is infectious.

So why do so many people volunteer?

Actually we recently conducted some research called Hidden Diamonds – specifically to look at the value of volunteering. Traditionally the value around volunteering was determined by working out how much it would cost to replace volunteers with paid staff. But we wanted to look at the softer benefits of 'what's in it for me?'

What we found is people who volunteer in sports in particular are happier and less likely to worry. They grow and develop skills, they make new friends, because sport's quite social, but also importantly they learn to trust their community better, because they're engaging with them in a different way than they would have done before. So they get to feel more like they're part of their community, they feel that they have more of an influence on their community, have more of a say. So volunteering is really good to develop both physical and mental well-being, as well as bringing the community together.

One of my highlights every December is attending the BBC Sports Personality of the Year party. Over the years, as well as elite sports people, I've been fortunate to meet and chat to several winners of the Unsung Hero award. This is given to someone nominated by the public, who devotes their free time to helping people in grass roots sports and fitness activities. Smiling, encouraging, mentoring and lifting spirits – winners are always dedicated to helping others in their communities or clubs. They're properly inspiring people. Chantel, unsurprisingly, agrees.

The Join In Trust also examined the behaviour behind volunteers. One of the things we found is that club sports just wouldn't take place or survive without volunteers. The average number of volunteers per grass-roots club in the UK is 24 and the average number of participants or members is 220. So that works out to each volunteer having the capacity to bring roughly nine participants into sport.

I know she's keen to start heading to France on her summer holidays, but Chantel's zeal is catching. I find myself thinking aloud how volunteering in sport is 360 degrees of awesome. Not only do the volunteers themselves gain benefits, they also help the nation become active. Which I guess is why Sport England is investing millions of pounds in volunteering. I ask Chantel if she knows how many people come into sport via volunteering.

We don't know at the moment, but that is exactly why Sport England is investing in sports volunteering, because we want to be able to put that label on it. And we want to know exactly how many people get active, physically active, in sport and recreation because of the role that a volunteer plays. I mean, we see it at a grass-roots level with volunteers. The more volunteers you have in a community, the more they're out and about and the more they're talking about volunteering, obviously it increases the number of volunteers.

Could more sport happen with more volunteers? Of course. So we want to make sure that grass-roots clubs and organisations that need volunteers are uncovering every stone. Typically they do a lot of their recruitment through word of mouth, and whilst that works to a degree, most clubs will say they need more volunteers. So perhaps other channels need to be explored.

But I suspect the only channel Chantel wants to explore at this moment is the English Channel on her way to France. I thank her and wish her *bon voyage*.

Back in the South Downs, thoughts turn wistfully to home and sleep. We begin packing all the equipment back into the wire container as we wait for the final runner. This involves another painful trip into the bush, but while I'm in there, cursing again as more skin ruptures, we hear word that the last competitor actually stopped some time ago so we're free to go. The lorry arrives and picks up the equipment ready for the next race – and the next set of eager volunteers who'll happily clamber through thorns to make runners' lives a little easier.

3. conwy

My wife has got it into her head that Crib Goch will be the death of me. Literally. That trying to cross this precariously narrow mountain ridge in Wales will do me in. That I'll fall down one of its 1,000-foot sheer sides and that'll be that.

Crib Goch – the name means 'red ridge' in Welsh – is a knife-edged arête (or ridge) near the summit of Mount Snowdon. It's about half a mile long. As well as being one of the most perilous places in the UK, it's also among the wettest, with average rainfall of 200 inches a year. It's one of the windiest spots too – as I can testify. Crosswinds of 40 miles an hour are buffeting me as I approach. Whilst running, I've been aiming slightly east of where I want to land and the wind's blown me back on course. Most people choose other routes up the tallest mountain in England and Wales.

The treacherous traverse of Crib Goch comes towards the end of the first day of the Dragon's Back Race, a world-renowned, multi-stage mountain race. Five days on remote, wild, trackless terrain along the mountainous spine of Wales, from the castle walls in the picturesque market town of Conwy on the north coast to the cosy village of Llandeilo in the far south. Climbing and clambering as much as running – 200 miles in total with over 50,000 feet of vertical ascent. By common consent, this is the world's toughest mountain race – which in my opinion puts it high in the reckoning for world's toughest multi-stage race, period.

By the time we reach Crib Goch, we've run further than a marathon and climbed the equivalent of three times up Mount Snowdon. Assuming we survive the ridge, an actual ascent of Snowdon will follow soon after.

My wonderful wife has been fretting about this moment ever since I entered five months ago. The first thing she saw on the Dragon's Back Race website was a photo of a competitor crossing this notorious ridge, its lethal potential glaring back unapologetically. And it didn't help that when she proceeded to type 'Crib Goch' into Google, one of the suggested popular searches was 'Crib Goch deaths'. She's truly brilliant, Caroline, and gorgeous – but she doesn't half worry. For almost half a year, the idea that Crib Goch could kill me has been firmly embedded in her head. And with all her anxiety and apprehension building to a race day crescendo, the same idea has begun seeping unsolicited into mine.

Especially now.

Now I've finally made it to the top of another strength-sapping climb and seen the ridge in person for the first time. It's one thing contemplating the traverse in theory, quite another when you witness those dizzying drops in person. And this wind! These ferocious, 40mph gusts aren't making me feel any more secure. Neither is the presence of a mountain rescue volunteer, who calmly suggests, 'Don't be a hero'. I mean, what does that even mean? How would you go about being a hero in the wind on Crib Goch? At the moment I'm seriously considering being the exact opposite and abandoning the race here and now. After all, I've got a young family to consider....

What am I doing up here anyway? I feel like an imposter, a fish out of water. A hippopotamus among mountain goats. I've never previously attempted a multi-stage race, or a mountain race, a self-navigation race, or indeed been in the mountains. Not properly anyway. My only previous foray into Wales came courtesy of the kindness of one of the pre-race favourites. Jez Bragg took me under his wing a few months previously. I knew of Jez after his victory in the iconic Ultra-Trail du Mont-Blanc (103 miles around Europe's tallest peak) when he was 29. He also held the record for the quickest Ramsay Round in Scotland (58 miles, 24 summits, 18 hours) and is the fastest man to run the length of New Zealand, completing the 2,000-mile Te Araroa Trail in just 53 days.

Jez got in touch out of the blue, an email to ask if I fancied a run together in Snowdonia. Did I ever! A chance to discover the Welsh mountains with an elite athlete, a man who'd been in contention to win the 2015 Dragon's Back Race before a vicious stomach bug, picked up when he drank from a mountain stream, stopped him violently in his tracks…. The offer even fills me with a tiny amount of confidence: Jez must think I'm competent enough not to be a complete waste of his time. Also, I'll have a far better chance of finishing the race if I know what I'm getting myself into. (As it turns out, Jez doesn't think I'm capable, quite the opposite in fact – he's doing a favour for the organisers who want to know what *they're* letting themselves in for, allowing me in!) We arrange to meet during the Easter holidays, when I'm by the seaside with the extended family; the Kent coast to Conwy during rush hour is a proper drive, let me tell you.

My lovely in-laws didn't bat an eyelid when I left our holiday cottage a day early to go running. Jez's in-laws though – off the scale. His wife's dad offered to drive us into the centre of Snowdonia at 5 o'clock in the morning. The plan was to attempt to replicate the first day's route with the help of the map Jez had kept from 2015. But when you're running 35 miles over a dozen mountains from Conwy to the foot of Snowdon, you need logistics. A car at the finishing point, and a fantastic father-in-law to drive you to the start before dawn.

The night before, Jez texted me the coordinates to a car park. A grid reference: SH627506. 'See you there!' he added cheerfully. I replied with a 'Great!' though I didn't have the faintest idea what he was talking about. SH627506? What the hell is that? I tried typing it into the map app of the iPhone. 'No results found'. There was absolutely no way I was going to admit my ignorance and request further directions, but at the same time I was slightly anxious about the following morning's rendezvous. Still, I could always call if I was struggling. Little did I know.

In London you're rarely without Wifi or 4G, even on the Underground. Worst-case scenario is the odd corner of frustratingly slow GPRS (whatever that means). In Snowdonia, there are huge expanses of Welsh countryside many, many miles across which have absolutely no phone signal at all. Zero. You may as well not have a phone. I actually think this is tremendous, but not in all circumstances. So when I set off in the dark with no clear idea where I was going, I wasn't nearly as worried as I should have been. I was largely guessing, and hoping the meeting point would be obvious. When it wasn't, and the full horror of the mobile reception situation hit home, I started to become uneasy. Which soon became jittery, and before long I had a case of the full-blown heebie-jeebies. No proper destination, and no way of getting in touch. Here was an elite ultra-runner who was giving up his day (his birthday, I would later discover) to run with me, who'd dragged his father-in-law out of bed at 4am to help – and there was every chance I'd never find him. To add to my worries, I was close to running out of petrol. There are no 24-hour petrol stations in this part of Wales either.

At five to five, five minutes early, I found a likely looking car park in the dark. No other cars about, no houses. Just a toilet and an old-fashioned phone box which only took coins – and I didn't have any. My best option, my least worst option, was to wait and hope. Within a minute, my heart leapt as car lights appeared in the distance, approached... and went past without slowing. Was that Jez on his way somewhere else? Should I follow? Bearing in mind the petrol warning light I decided to stay put. After that nothing happened for 15 minutes. Apart from those heebie-jeebies having kittens.

Extraordinary how powerless you feel without a phone these days. For every second of those long minutes, almost 1,000 of them, all I could think about was how the horror of this morning would haunt me all the way to the start line. And then Jez turned up.

He'd had a bit of a morning too. His father-in-law had spent the night throwing up so he'd come on his own but was increasingly concerned about running out of diesel.

We hastily devised a new plan. Drive my car to Conwy, find a petrol station, fill both it and a jerrycan, park up and run the race route over the mountains back to SH627506 – from where Jez could drive me back to my car. It says a lot about our nervous states that we didn't spot the obvious fly in the ointment – namely that we'd have to run for a whole day over mountains, including a traverse of Crib Goch, carrying five litres of diesel.

It still didn't dawn on us, the jerrycan sitting uselessly in the boot of my car, when we set off from the ruins of Conwy Castle, as the race would do five weeks later. Up Conwy Mountain we jogged. Everything was going smoothly when suddenly, to my astonishment, the paths ran out.

I'd been expecting the countryside to be a gnarlier version of Richmond Park. Steeper and hillier certainly, and bigger, more beautiful, more remote – but still largely... tame. We were in the UK after all. I simply didn't know this sort of stuff existed here. I tried to remember back to my weekend running in the Lake District – both the Keswick Half Marathon and my own explores followed pathways. Here though? No phone signal, now no footpaths; I was way out of my comfort zone.

By contrast Jez comes to Snowdonia a lot, owns a house here, trains here most weeks, and he found my surprise both endearing and frustrating. I hesitated as I watched him run through a bog, expecting me to follow. I opted to skirt around instead. Baffled, he shook his head. 'You're only delaying the inevitable,' he advised. 'Your feet are permanently wet when you run up here.'

'We'll see about that,' I thought. About a minute later, I realised he was right as I squelched through a large expanse of standing water. Even running around it wouldn't solve the problem. Wet feet and Welsh mountains simply go together. There's no other option. Thanks to the lack of paths, you have the choice of the entire landscape – and most of it's wet. Short grass, long grass up to your shins, heather. Also rocks of all sizes, sometimes nestled into the hillside or more usually in clusters – and they can be lethally slippery. If you do find the occasional cattle trod to follow, a thin line of shorter grass where animals have chosen to walk, you consider that a win as you open your stride. But even trods can be splashy. The terrain is very unforgiving, and requires your permanent attention. Three hours into our run, I'd almost fallen over lots of times and actually fallen over five times. Jez lost his footing on a rock once, but recovered easily.

I decided to ask him how wild our current terrain is on a scale of one to 10. Given the lack of any obvious evidence that humans had ever been here before us, I was expecting a nine or a 10.

'Five or six,' came the jaunty reply. 'Just wait until we reach the... hang on, where's my phone?'

Jez had lost his phone. He'd been taking scenic selfies about an hour earlier when we stopped for some snacks (I'd brought a packet of fruits, nuts and seeds, he had energy bars) and he didn't replace the phone securely enough in his running pack. We had no option but to retrace our steps, a task that would've been a hell of a lot easier if there had been footpaths to follow.

We crested a peak, and I chanced a glance at my own phone. Hallelujah! One heavenly bar of mobile signal! Jez swiftly signed in to his Apple account before the reception disappeared, and we followed a small blue dot on the screen all the way back to his phone. No paths or people up here – but no problem using Find My iPhone to recover a lost mobile.

By this time there was no way of making it back to his car in daylight, and the diesel situation had finally dawned on us too. So we decided to return to Conwy and drive back to his car (via the local Tesco to buy Jez a birthday cake). It turns out SH627506 is at the foot of Mount Snowdon with a well-trodden route (the Watkin Path – an actual path!) to the top. There were still several hours of daylight left, so we thought we'd nip to the summit before Jez returned to a sickly father-in-law and a birthday dinner whilst I braved the bank holiday traffic back to Kent.

We went at our own pace, so within minutes Jez had disappeared into the clag* and that was the last I saw of him until the official Dragon's Back Race briefing the night before the race.

---

* 'Clag' is a mountain runners' term for bad weather around a peak. It usually means poor visibility due to cloud, and often involves damp and general misery. The word 'clag' gets used a lot. If you're ever stuck for something to say around a mountain runner, just keep repeating the word 'clag' and watch them nod solemnly.

If I'd been feeling nervous beforehand, the briefing does little to cheer me up. Shane Ohly is the man in charge, and he seems to delight in accentuating the difficulties that lie in store. Some of the advice/ instruction that sticks is: 'Drink from any stream you like, but not from beneath the farm line', and 'If you're in imminent danger of death, press your emergency button. But only if you're in actual imminent danger of death. If not, you have a map and two legs – so please just sort yourself out.'

The assembled runners look fit, experienced and most of all – capable. My usual method of *turn up and see how it goes* has no place here. Like I say, I feel like an imposter.

The race rules are simple. You have a map with a suggested route highlighted, but you're under no obligation to follow it. All you have to do is check in ('dib in', via a small plastic GPS tracker attached permanently to your wrist) at various checkpoints along the way, around 20 of them each day, and reach the campsite at the finish by 11pm each evening. The checkpoints are small boxes which tend to be located on mountain peaks. They prevent anyone taking short cuts or missing any climbing. You're entirely self-sufficient, carrying all your own water, food and clothing for the day – although they do let you refill water bottles and restock supplies at a prearranged 'drop bag point' around two-thirds of the way through the day. You leave a small bag (5kg or under, and they do weigh it, which must be waterproof, as this is Wales) as you set off in the morning, and it'll be waiting for you when you reach the designated rendezvous. There's a suggested latest time to arrive at each checkpoint, and an actual cut-off time at the drop bag point – one second late here, and you're pulled from the race. The accepted wisdom is to follow the map as closely as possible unless you're a mountain veteran or a genius.

This is all very new to me, and nerve-wracking. I'd taught myself how to read a map, via the FAQ on the Ordnance Survey website, on the train to Conwy that morning. To add to my worries, a phone call from home.

'Did you definitely pack your watch charging lead?'

'Yes, no question. It was the last thing I put into my bag. Why?'

'I've just found something that looks suspiciously like your Garmin lead in Mary's cot.'

Ah. So our youngest had been at my kit bag as I bade farewell to the others. Sub-optimal, to say the least. I was so freaked out by the prospect of losing the ability to use my GPS watch that I even called our local minicab firm in Barnes, SW London, to ask how much to deliver the lead 250 miles to Conwy overnight. It was a short conversation (£300!) so my only option was to find someone else using the new Fenix 5X – and beg to borrow their lead during the race.

And so it was that as everyone else lined up in the castle ruins for the ceremonial start, waving up at photographers on the ramparts, I was shuffling around the assembled runners staring at wrists.

'Excuse me, is that the Garmin Fenix?'

'No it's a Forerunner, why?'

'Don't worry, have a good race…. Excuse me, is that a Fenix…?'

As it turns out, the Fenix 3, which almost everybody has, and the new Fenix 5, which nobody but me seems to have, use different charging leads, but look almost identical. A Welsh male voice choir serenades the runners in the castle. This is something I'd been looking forward to, a perfect way to begin a race spanning the entire length of the country. But I'm still moving around furtively in the crowd of runners, staring at wrists.

'Excuse me, is that a Fenix 5?'

Suddenly the countdown begins and we're away. These are the first steps I've run for a fortnight. My right ankle's been playing up and I've been advised to give the injury – a 'high ankle sprain' – maximum chance to recover. Probably best not to recall too closely the conversation I had with my physio when I told him what race I was planning to put my injured ankle through.

Bloody stupid way to get injured, too. A day at Box Hill in Surrey with the family, and I took the opportunity to get a few hill reps in. Halfway up the first one I wondered how long I'd been running, glanced at my watch and next thing I knew, I was on the floor regaining consciousness. I'd managed to knock myself out on a low-hanging tree branch. Having checked my stopwatch just before the unfortunate accident, I could accurately estimate that I'd been out for 10 seconds. More worryingly, though I didn't know it yet, I'd landed awkwardly on my ankle and sprained it badly. I gingerly continued running, trying to remember the advice about running and concussion, and as I passed my family on what I hoped would be the first of five or six loops, my attention was drawn to the sight of my son flying upwards through the air.

Only a 10-year-old boy can contrive to break his hand like our Matthew broke his hand that day. He'd fashioned a see-saw out of two enormous bits of wood, positioned himself on the low end of the lever and asked his biggest cousin to jump from a tree onto the high side. The purpose was to see how far skywards Matthew could be launched – and in that respect the exercise was a huge success. The trouble came as he returned to earth and managed to trap his hand between the two huge lumps of wood.

So I didn't really give my own growing, nagging ankle pain much thought until after we'd left A&E much later that evening, with Matthew's hand in bandages. He was cursing the fact that he'd broken his left hand (so would still have to do his homework but wouldn't be able to play football or go diving) when I first thought something might be up with my right foot. I ignored it, in the truest tradition of runners burying their heads in the sand about possible injuries, and continued to run on it. It only started becoming something I couldn't ignore as I began a self-devised treadmill hill-training regime to try to get some much-needed mountain strength into my soft London legs (25kg in a rucksack, treadmill on max incline, go as fast as possible for an hour – I have no idea if it did any good, but nothing I've ever done before or since has made me sweat so profusely). Several trips to the physio, and plenty of ice and ibuprofen later, and the ankle is rested, strapped and (hopefully) ready for the rigours to come.

It gives an ominous growl of umbrage as I start running slowly around the castle ramparts. What with the pain coming from below, and the ongoing panic about charging my watch, it's a real effort to drag my attention back to the race itself, to this spectacular start. One loop of the castle, and it's time to 'dib in' for the first time. Checkpoint 1, completed. Next stop, Checkpoint 2 on the summit of Conwy Mountain.

The following few hours are entirely pleasant. We climb, descend and run along ridges. Lots of chatting, meeting new people, making new friends. Interspersed with the odd torpedo of pain every time I twist my right ankle on a loose stone or boulder. I remember to eat most hours (I've got loads of bars with me – oat, energy and chocolate) and to take frequent sips from the Evian bottles bulging out of the front pockets of my running pack. This is tough, but fun. I hold my own when there's flat or uphill running to be done, even when there's scrambling or climbing ('technical sections', the diehards call them). But on the descents I struggle.

I honestly don't know whether I'd fare any better without an injured ankle. Certainly trying to protect it can't help, and I'm at my most cautious when the gradient goes downwards. But by the same token, even fully fit I wouldn't have the skill, or the bravery, of many of those around me. They seem to fly down these wild mountains as if they're skipping downstairs for breakfast. It's terrific to watch.

Checkpoints come and go, and then we run around a large, spectacular mountaintop horseshoe – this is proper runnable terrain, relatively little danger to my ankle, and I make the most of it. The only issue is the fierce wind – not unusual up here, I'm told. It's a sidewind and it's so strong, you have to aim slightly off in order to run straight. The breeze blows you back on course. It's disconcerting, but kind of cool.

Eventually we reach a long, difficult, 'technical' descent to the valley below. Running implies a maximum of one contact point with the ground. Now I mostly have three, four, sometimes five. I'm using hands, elbows, bottom, even chin. There are huge boulders strewn across the mountain, often with big gaps between them. The only way down is to sit on one massive grey stone, tentatively reach out for the next with your leg, and lower yourself onto it with your arms. I feel guilty as more adept competitors are forced to wait behind me; this is the only way down and there's nowhere to move aside.

I remember back to Jez telling me that the slopes above Conwy were no more than five or six out of 10 on the wilderness scale. I ask the bloke behind me if this counts as a 10. Surely this is as bad as it can get?

He shakes his head in what I suspect to be a pitying, patronising kind of way, and splashes through a huge puddle as he finds a place to finally get past. The enticing ribbon lake Llyn Ogwen below never seems to get any closer. The descent takes an hour, which feels like three.

Finally we reach level ground and – special treat! – some tarmac. I revel in the road's fast, flat surface. It's only for half a mile or so as we run around the reservoir towards the day's drop bag point in a convenient car park, but this concentration-free running is sheer bliss. You don't realise how much it takes out of you when you're having to focus on every footstep. Just for the hell of it, I overtake three or four others who are sensibly conserving energy.

Every drop bag point has a cut-off time attached to it. I'm thrilled to discover I'm hours ahead of schedule as I'm handed the new lime green drybag I purchased especially four days ago. Inside, though I can't remember buying it, is a packet of pork scratchings. I was once told by a very clever doctor that pork scratchings are the one food with absolutely no nutritional value at all. Everything you're putting in your mouth is the bad stuff. Well, that doctor has obviously never tried a bag of pork scratchings in the middle of a mountain ultra. The salt, the fat, the crunch. I can't ever remember enjoying eating something more.

A refill of the water bottles, and it's time for what I'm told is one of three proper climbs between here and the campsite. A daddy climb, a mummy climb and a baby climb. This is apparently the baby. But bloody hell it goes on forever. The celebrated mountain running photographer and writer, Ian Corless, meets us with his camera on what I assume to be the summit, but what turns out to be about halfway up. This is Tryfan we're climbing, just over 3,000 feet high and you definitely wouldn't mistake it for anything but a mountain. It has that classic pointy shape, and twin monoliths, two giant pillar-like boulders ('Adam' and 'Eve') on the top. Those who jump from one to the other, apart from being soft in the head on a day like this, are said to gain the 'Freedom of Tryfan'. I'm very pleased to hear the reassuring bleep as I point my wrist at the little box. Checkpoint 12.

Checkpoint 13, on the slightly higher summit of Glyder Fach, the sixth highest in Wales, is no more than a mile away – but it takes almost an hour to get there. As does the top of Glyder Fawr, the fifth highest peak and Checkpoint 14. The going is properly rocky, enormous boulders jutting out of the countryside like some giant hand has scattered them from the sky. It's not just me: nobody seems to be especially quick over this stuff. The scenery though, gosh. Every time you feel frustrated at the slow-going, just look up. Or rather, look down and around. The sun's out and you can see for miles in all directions. Large lakes below look like puddles, above them vast curving grey rockfaces stained here and there by dark green moss. The sheer scale and solitude of the place is deeply impressive. All day, I hardly see a soul who's not connected to the race.

Four of us are together as we make the descent to the youth hostel at Pen-y-Pass. We pause to grab a quick round of Cokes for energy. The atmosphere is one of nervous excitement. With the emphasis on nervous. There's no putting this off. Crib Goch is next.

4. keswick

Two years previously, Jasmin Paris was third in the Dragon's Back Race as she reached Pen-y-Pass and started up the Pyg Track towards Crib Goch. She didn't hesitate, buy a fizzy drink, overthink or worry. She simply reached the ridge and skipped over it like the drop on either side was less than a foot, rather than over a thousand. Four days later, she went on to win the women's race and finish second overall. The way she tells it, Jim Mann (a good friend of hers) only beat her because she let him.

I've chatted to Jasmin several times on the phone, but I've never met her. Even so, as my phone randomly receives reception while I'm buying Cokes in the hostel and beeps to let me know I have a message, I check to see a text from Jasmin wishing me luck for the week. They really are a first-rate bunch of people, fell runners.

We'd first spoken 11 months previously when she'd broken the record for the Ramsay Round in Scotland, a circuit of 58 miles, taking in 24 summits including Ben Nevis, with a total climb of around 28,000 feet. Two months before that, she'd obliterated the women's record for the more famous Bob Graham Round in the Lake District, taking two and a half hours off the previous mark set by her pal Nicky Spinks. Starting and finishing at the Moot Hall in Keswick, you need to climb the 42 peaks (encompassing 27,000 feet of climbing and 66 miles of running) inside 24 hours to gain entry to the Bob Graham Club. Many more people fail than succeed. Jasmin's time was 15:24. She would also break the record for the Paddy Buckley Round (47 summits in Snowdonia) later that same year. Her Ramsay record is not just a women's record, but an overall Fastest Known Time for the route. As you can imagine, she was suddenly the centre of attention.

Yes, after the Bob Graham I was quite taken aback because it was such a media storm. I guess the furthest waves of that reached into the more general media, like the *Guardian* or BBC Radio 2. In terms of fell running circles as well, it went completely wild. I guess for me, it's not that I wanted to be famous. In fact, that's not me at all. I'm not particularly bothered about being famous and recognised.

It's more the idea that I could inspire people to do things. People have said to me, 'Listening to you has made me want to go out and explore the Highlands more' or, 'I think I'm going to give this a go' – I find that really wonderful. It's a really positive thing – quite unexpected, but incredible.

In terms of women and sport, I love the fact that you can believe in yourself and push the boundaries. Because I think fell running is really quite genderless in the sense that women race against men. When I race, I don't really consider who I'm racing against, if there's a man next to me or a woman. You just race because you're racing against the person who's going similarly fast. It's nice that ultimately the achievements of myself and Nicky have shown that women have an equal place in sport and in fell running and in the mountains.

The extraordinary thing about Jasmin Paris, one of the many, is that she doesn't really consider herself an athlete first and foremost. I once met Roger Bannister, the first man to run a mile in under four minutes. At the time, in 1954, it was major world news. But on the 50th anniversary of his achievement – still one of the greatest ever by a British athlete – he told me he's prouder of his subsequent accomplishments in the medical field and that his athletic endeavours are secondary. Jasmin, I think, feels the same. As well as running, she's doing important research into finding cures for cancer.

I'd like to feel I can make a contribution to science that's going to make a difference long-term. I know that for me, my career is really important. There's no way that I would give up what I do to become a sponsored, full-time athlete. I have been asked, but there's just no way I would do it.

And I do think that running is just a hobby. I sort of feel that these are fun achievements and I'm really lucky to be able to do it at all. It's more that I'm just having fun and I happen to be good at it. And I think what I do in science is more serious and more important.

It's also time-consuming, frequently requiring 12-hour days – leaving home at seven in the morning and not returning until 6 or 7pm. How on earth does she fit in her training?

I get up most days at five and run for, like, an hour, an hour and a half before work. And I also sometimes do some swimming or go to the gym in the evening – so I sort of double train. I never particularly have any sort of strict regime planned out beforehand. When I can do something twice a day, I feel like that's probably good.

Running-wise, during the week, just an hour, an hour and a half every day and that's always in the hills. Then at weekends, long distance – probably on average four hours on both Saturday and Sunday, again on the hills. Big days out on the hills.

It's not hard to motivate myself to get up at five to run. I really enjoy being out. I never, ever get back from a run and regret having gone. We live in a really lovely area so I run straight from the house, right into hills. And I enjoy the feeling of running. Even in the winter, you go out and see owls, foxes and deer. It's still really beautiful, even if you're running at night.

However, at the end of last season when I was pretty tired and I'd done all the big things that I wanted to do, I suddenly found it much harder to motivate myself.

Jasmin also started running relatively late, after she left university. She was working as a local vet and somebody suggested she start running. She went along to a fell race, and was hooked.

I did a bit of running before that but it was more the sort of run around the park, a 15-, 20-minute thing. It wasn't until I did that first fell race that

I thought, 'This is fantastic!' The combination of being in the hills and running. Also the discovery of all these people who are similarly minded to me, who wanted to run for fun's sake.

It's a very open community, very friendly. Even racing, championship racing, the elite runners will be racing with the slowest runners, and there's no distinction. When you're lined up for your tea and cake at the end there's absolutely no elitism in this sport. It's lovely. It's so welcoming to anyone, and I think that goes hand in hand with the ethos of being outdoors in the mountains.

I meet people all the time who are really interesting, who enjoy nature and the outdoors and have similar outlooks on the world really. Now as a runner, I do feel like you have this urge, you want to go for a run every day.

Those three record-breaking rounds of hers, they all came within a few months of each other. She ranks the Ramsay record as the greatest achievement – not just because she also broke the men's record, but because it's a horrendous logistical challenge. You always have people running with you on challenges like this, your supporters, carrying kit and food as well as verifying that all peaks have been accounted for. There are only three legs in a Ramsay Round (compared to five in a Bob Graham) so supporters have necessarily longer shifts and have to be highly accomplished runners themselves. The route doesn't cross a road, so they've already run several miles before they meet you. And the terrain is wilder; there's very little short runnable grass. For these reasons, fewer than 100 people have ever completed a Ramsay Round.

For Jasmin, the whole day went pretty much perfectly according to plan in Scotland. With a close-knit team of super-supporters around her and fuelled by confidence from her exploits in the Lakes, Jasmin always knew she was gunning for the Fastest Known Time (FKT). And she absolutely smashed it. Then straight to the pub for a burger and chips and one solitary pint of beer before falling asleep.

The Ramsay Record is the one she'd choose if she could only take one to a desert island, but she's incredibly loquacious when describing the Bob Graham day.

It's 4am and I'm in Steve Birkinshaw's house near Keswick, which I've borrowed as a base for all my supporters. Steve set the record for the Wainwright's Round (214 Lakeland Peaks). So everyone gathered at Steve's the night before and it was a really good atmosphere. Basically we were all drinking tea and eating cake and chatting.

We eventually go to bed, but have to be up really early to start at the Moot Hall at 4am. We set off up Skiddaw. I have no pack, obviously, because it's being carried for me. I've also recently recovered from a bad case of food poisoning, so for a few weeks I've had this enforced taper as I couldn't really do much running while I was sick… which is actually really good because I'm not very good at tapering. So I'm well rested and I'm running without a pack. And I'm fit. It feels like I can just fly. I could run all the way up that first mountain and I'm constantly being told to slow down, slow down… and then we reach the summit and we're fully 10 minutes ahead of schedule. I'm just amazed because it feels so easy.

As we come off Skiddaw and I start to climb Calva, it begins to get light. By the time we come up Blencathra, it's dawn and the sky is full of orange and purple. Stunning. And then we're down the steep drop into the changeover place, and I lose half of my support team because they can't keep up so I'm down to one person.

The second leg is when I distinctly feel like I can simply run for ever. We're on that Helvellyn Ridge and it's frosty, and the sun is sparkling off the dew on the grass. It's easy running and I'm feeling good and yeah, it's pretty special. And then coming into the changeover for the leg three, which is that long leg, and I'm beginning to tire. But then this is also my favourite mountain running, Scafell and that rocky section, then down into Wasdale.

In the fourth leg, I'm quite tired, but by the time we get towards the end of it everyone is feeling pretty jubilant because we think I've basically cracked it. We knew it was going to be good. And the final leg, going over those three final peaks, Dale Head, Hindscarth, Robinson, we're like a big social party because all the people from previous legs come back and join in again. The pace isn't that fast any more, I think everybody is just having a really good time. I'm not actually doing that much talking by now, but the others are all chattering away.

Then running into the final section, into Keswick, is quite amazing because there's this event going on at the Moot Hall (where the Round begins and ends). There are loads of people going on a charity walk up Cat Bells with head torches, 'Lighting Up Cat Bells for Nepal' it's called. So there are about 300 people coincidentally gathered outside the hall. They have nothing to do with me. But my support team put the word out that I'm about to arrive and need to be able to get through – and the crowd really gets behind me. Hundreds of people all come running down towards Moot Hall, then the crowd parts and I run through this huge crowd of cheering, clapping people with photographers and everything. It makes the end even more memorable because, you know, that was a pretty good atmosphere. And then just hugs and the pub for a burger and beer.

The previous holder of the women's record in both rounds, the Bob Graham and the Ramsay, is Nicky Spinks, a farmer from Yorkshire. She's quite sanguine about losing those records relatively soon after breaking them.

Yeah, I know Jasmin's gone after me. I haven't held the records very long and she's gone and broken them, but she's absolutely whooped my butt really. In a way it's better that she's done that. I got to where I was through hard work and organisation, but she's actually got loads of talent to add to the organisation and hard work. So she's put the bar really high, but it's where it should be now I think.

There's a tremendous tradition in fell running of existing record holders helping others break their records. So whilst you might expect Jasmin Paris and Nicky Spinks to be rivals, actually quite the opposite is true. As Jasmin says:

I wouldn't consider myself a rival of Nicky in any way. When I set out to run the rounds, it's because I really wanted to see how well I could do them. It wasn't so much with the aim of beating all three ladies' records. So breaking Nicky's records was kind of a little bit of a side issue. In shorter races I'm faster than Nicky and I think we both know that so we don't race against each other in fell races and go head-to-head on a week-to-week basis.

We're good friends really. I supported her Bob Graham and actually, when she ran the double I ran three of the 10 legs with her. And then her Ramsay Round, I supported that too. It's a mutual friendship. She came out to the UTMB* as well this year and stayed with our family in the chalet so yeah, I think we're friends.

Anyway I can't break her most recent record for 17 years because it was an over fifties challenge. I think that's actually why she ran it. She set the record on her 50th birthday.

It's only a few weeks after Nicky Spinks' 50th birthday when I catch up with her. She's just back from a run with the juniors she coaches. You can tell she's still thrilled by how well it went.

It was a lovely evening. So driving to the club I was thinking, 'Oh what should we do?' I'm always trying to encourage them onto the fells, but it's

---

* Ultra-Trail du Mont-Blanc. The most iconic mountain race on the calendar, held in late August. Starting and finishing in Chamonix, 2,000 runners follow the Tour du Mont Blanc through France, Italy and Switzerland for 103 miles with 31,500 feet of climbing. In between breaking all three Rounds records in 2016, Jasmin finished sixth.

41

in Penistone so we can't get to the fells easily. But there's Hartcliff Hill and I was thinking, 'Well, maybe we could just get them out there.'

I ran them along a road, they're pretty good teenagers, there's about eight of them. We get them to this hill and there's only a couple complaining. But then we reach the top and sit down and there's this little patch of heather, it was like being on the moors. And looking out across the moorland you could see for miles. They were all like, 'Wow!'

They actually asked me to take photos, and I do love it if I can encourage them, especially the young. This is why we've just run all the way up this long horrible hill, to get here to look at the view and now we can run down a lovely footpath all the way back again. A really great evening.

It's not just the young runners of South Yorkshire who are inspired by Nicky Spinks. I am too, as are countless others who enjoy running in the fells. And she's a paragon of hope for women with breast cancer. In 2005 she was diagnosed with a tumour, and hopes her subsequent exploits reassure and embolden women who are going through the same. It's one of the reasons she attempted – and broke – the record for the scarcely credible double Bob Graham Round.

When I got breast cancer, I was looking online and there's more tales of people that haven't lived than people that have lived. In fact I think there are more people that do survive, it's just that they don't go on the Internet and say, 'I've lived.'

So I did want to get my name out there and hope someone with cancer can look at my picture and go, 'Well, she lived 10 years then I might be able to as well.' When I was ill I found a little picture of a woman who was a trustee of a charity, and I printed it off and whenever I was feeling down I used to look at her and just think, 'She lived 10 years, maybe I will.'

Eleven years after her cancer diagnosis, Nicky completed her double Bob Graham Round. It took her 46 hours to complete. Almost two solid days' running on tricky terrain. What on earth is that like?

It's continuous. I broke it down into 30 hours, which was from the Moot Hall out to Yewbarrow and back again. I assumed I would be strong enough to just go out and do another 16 on top of that. But going through Keswick was pretty hard because I wasn't feeling great. I couldn't face going out and doing another 16 hours, but I had a power nap, which sorted me out. It was strange to run for that long, especially doing two laps because as you're going out and you've been running for four hours, say, you're chatting with your support about what you'll do here next time – and then you realise that that won't be for another 20 hours!

But I know I'm so stubborn – if I don't get round, I'll just come back and do it all over again. So I might as well try to sort out whatever's going wrong and finish it this time. Do it now, you don't have to come back and do it again. I'm really strict with myself when I'm running; the rules are the rules. I think I can put myself through quite a lot of discomfort to achieve what I want to achieve. And I'm better now at sorting myself out as I'm running so that I don't get as many dips in energy and mood levels. It's really about making yourself eat every hour and a half so you don't get that dip in energy where everything is falling. Also I cut it all down so if I've got a schedule or a map I don't look at all of it. Just fold it all up so you only see the bit you're on.

When we finished and broke the record, I never even managed to get to the pub. It was about half nine, we had a couple of drinks at the Moot Hall but then I really desperately needed to sleep, so we just went back to the camp site. But I managed to lock my keys in the van. So I had to sleep in a friend's van while she called the breakdown people and they all tried to break into my van.

Like Jasmin Paris, Nicky didn't always run. Not like this anyway. She ran around her parents' farm in Derbyshire as a kid, but she put much of her athletic ability at school (she generally beat her classmates in races) down to the fact that 'farm kids run better'. Then as an adult, for many years she just ran three times a week 'to keep the weight down'.

I got into it again in 2001, when a friend was doing a local parkrun, Leeds Abbey Dash. From there it went 10K, half marathon and then I found off-road running, trail races. And I knew once I'd found trail races, I wouldn't want to do roads again. They're just more interesting, not as boring as road because you've got to watch where your feet are going. Thinking about that, it takes your mind off things, and adds an extra dimension. And the terrain is constantly changing so you're also changing your gait, and your breathing, and having to pick your feet up.

Now it feels like it's time that women come forward more because we're only just behind the men. It wasn't until the mid-70s that we were allowed to even run marathons. We're 30 years behind the men in terms of women knowing that they can do this sort of thing. There are so many women who don't give things a go because they don't think they're going to be any good, or they haven't got the confidence.

I would say look at people like me and Jasmin. I was just a mid-pack runner when I first started. First time I did Wasdale*, I was like everybody else and just wanted to get around. You concentrate on what you're good at and get better at what you're not good at. And go slowly as well. I certainly didn't go from doing a 10K to a double Bob Graham; it's taken years.

People often pick something that's too far out of their reach, and then obviously they don't succeed and think they're no good. If I was going to give people advice, especially women, I'd say you need to go from a half marathon to a full marathon and then a 30-mile race and then something like a 60-miler. Pick things that have reasonable cut-offs, like the Long Distance Walkers Association. A lot of them welcome runners and obviously the cut-offs are do-able because they're for walkers – but they're great events and have great food, great organisation and they're really cheap.

---

* Wasdale Fell Race is held every July in the Lake District. About 21 miles long, with 9,000 feet of ascent. Some of the route is very rough, with steep technical ground and boulder fields.

Meanwhile, at the record-breaking end of fell running, was she not at least a little sad to see her records broken so swiftly, one after the other?

I think when Jasmin first got the Bob Graham I was like, 'Oh that's a bit sad.' Mainly because I'd only held it for a year or so. I think if I'd held it for longer it would have been a little bit easier, but then after that, when she went for the Ramsay and the Paddy Buckley, I actually started getting interested in how much she could take off. I've done my best, let's see what Jasmin can do with her best, which will be the record. Now, when people talk about the double Bob Graham record, I don't really see it as a record. It's just a long course with my time on it.

5. snowdon

The ascent to Crib Goch begins on a path called the Pyg Track. It's a gentle, clearly marked route, which I mostly take at a slow run or steady hike, depending on the gradient. The views all around are stunning – even after eight hours' slog in Snowdonia, the scenery doesn't get old. As I climb, I decide this is exactly the sort of path I'd enjoy returning to with my children*. The lakes Llyn Peris and Llyn Padarn appear in the far side of a U-shaped valley which itself was carved out at the end of the last Ice Age. I find myself wondering when these rocks were first trodden by human feet.

A signpost and the path forks. Another lake, Llyn Llydaw, the coldest in Britain, comes into sight below and the slopes of Y Lliwedd rise regally above the far side of the dark waters. The sign is red and written in forbidding capital letters: RHYBUDD FFORDD I CRIB GOCH. CAUTION ROUTE TO CRIB GOCH. Turn left for Snowdon summit the normal way; turn right for the ridge. A brief moment's hesitation – turning left means instant disqualification – and I do turn right.

The route from here becomes a full-on scramble. The next half-hour requires full concentration. It's not exposed up here but as a mountain novice, I'm definitely erring on the side of careful. The last 200 metres

---

* I did return with the family several months later, staying at the same hotel where Edmund Hillary and Tenzing Norgay trained for the first successful ascent of Mount Everest in 1953. Back in the day, the queue for the Pen-y-Gwryd bar would stretch out of the window and back in through the front door. They now have a ceremony for children under 13 who climb and descend Snowdon whilst staying at the hotel. The kids get to drink a celebratory Vimto from the very beaker Hillary took up Everest. Our elder two, Emily and Matthew, were thrilled to add their names to the roll of honour after making the ascent during the tail end of Storm Brian. Mary, three, is planning her Snowdon summit bid for the near future.

are climbed virtually straight upwards, and for the first time ever on a 'run' my arms start to ache.

All the while I've been chatting to someone who's essentially the exact opposite of a mountain novice. A fellow competitor, he's one of only a few hundred people in history to have scaled the so-called Seven Summits, the highest peaks on each of the seven continents: Everest, Aconcagua, Denali, Kilimanjaro, Elbrus, Puncak Jaya, Vinson. I'm continually asking him about Everest (the logistics, the difficulties, base camp, the traffic jam just below the summit), but he's much keener to discuss the hardest to climb of the seven, Puncak Jaya, which rises mysteriously from the dense tropical jungle of West Papua. I'm deeply impressed, whilst also continually calling him Jim, which I later learn to my embarrassment is not his name, it's John.

Jim (John) senses my apprehension as Crib Goch unfolds before us. He can tell I'm nervous and offers to help nurse me across. As an experienced mountaineer, traverses like this are doubtless meat and drink to him, and this is where he'd expect to make up time. And on the first afternoon of a five-day multi-stage ultra, time is absolutely key. The quicker you get back to camp, the quicker you can eat, prepare, sleep and recover – and the greater your chance of completing the following day. Left to his own devices, I'm sure John would stride happily over the apex of the arête. Thousand-foot drops don't hold much fear for someone who's climbed the Seven Summits. However, plain old niceness prevails – and John says he'll lead me across the easy way, just off to the left using the top of the ridge as a handrail. The wind, gusting up to 40mph, is blowing us mercifully into the rock face.

As we inch across, another Dragon's Back runner, a Swiss, races back towards us from the direction we're heading. He's on top of the ridge, jogging lightly and muttering to himself as he goes. It turns out he's forgotten to 'dib in' at the checkpoint box just before the start of Crib Goch. He's already fully crossed the ridge once, reached the next checkpoint on the other side, realised his error and he's now midway through a high speed reverse traverse, almost stepping on our fingers as he races back. Shortly afterwards, our fingertips are in danger again as our Swiss friend trots across the top of the ridge for a third time, having rectified his mistake. He's remarkably cheerful about it. Not to mention brave.

Seeing someone treat Crib Goch with such foolhardy abandon significantly lessens my fear, and John and I speed up. I even begin to enjoy myself up there – there's nothing like an exposed, windswept ridge to make you feel alive – and all too soon it's behind us. The only part of the week I was genuinely afraid about, and suddenly it's over, in the past. Yet there's so much of the race still to come. It feels like the men's 100 metres final at the Olympics coming on just the second evening of athletics: the blue riband event, but a bit too early.

But just like the Olympics, the sense of anti-climax doesn't last long. We're now on the summit of Garnedd Ugain, the second highest point in Wales and only 20 metres shorter than its more illustrious neighbour. Soon we join the final section of the Llanberis Path, the most popular and easiest hiking route up Snowdon – aka the Motorway. The Snowdon railway runs alongside. It's the perfect opportunity to remove the phone from its home inside a nappy bag in my rucksack (I get through a lot of nappy sacks whilst running; they're the perfect size to fit an iPhone and also perfectly waterproof). I still have reception, and get a text away to Caroline to let her know I'm over Crib Goch safely. I don't receive any reply as the phone signal promptly disappears, but I don't need one. Tidal waves of relief reach Snowdon from South West London through the ether.

No more than 10 minutes jogging up the Llanberis Path later, and we're on the summit of Snowdon. On a clear day, 18 lakes and 14 peaks over 3,000ft can be viewed from up here. Sometimes you can see as far as Ireland, the Isle of Man and the Lake District. But it's clouded over. Not that I mind. This isn't the time to stop and admire the views. I'm suddenly tired, and keen to finish and rest. I 'dib in' at the summit checkpoint and get on with it.

I know, because I've just been told, that there's still another few hours' hard graft around the Snowdon horseshoe before we reach the campsite. However, I also know, because I met Jez Bragg at grid reference SH627506 several weeks ago, that the campsite is currently very close by. In fact, the car park at SH627506 is just a few hundred yards from today's destination. Which means it's just a 45-minute hop from the top of Snowdon down the relatively straightforward Watkin Path, the first designated footpath in Britain. It was officially opened in 1892 by the 83-year-old Prime Minister, William Gladstone. He addressed a crowd of over 2,000 from a rock on the side of the path, known today as the Gladstone Rock. The Watkin Path was the first step towards opening the countryside to walkers.

There's some loose scree at the top of it and I almost fall as I peer down to see if the campsite is visible from up here. Soon the race route veers stubbornly off the Watkin Path towards more 'technical terrain'. This is where we begin our exacting tour of the Snowdon horseshoe. I'm getting used to the lingo by now – technical means 'un-runnable' and frequently involves using hands and arms as well as legs and feet. My injured right ankle is complaining loudly every time I twist or jar it, which on this terrain is every few seconds.

I misjudge one such footstep from one huge boulder to another and the pain is so severe I cry out in agony and collapse to the rocky floor. A fellow Dragon's Back runner hears and turns to help, hurrying 100 yards back over scraggy ground to check if I'm OK. By the time he reaches me I'm standing again, but limping severely. Once again I'm blown away by an act of kindness. Without a fuss, and without waiting to give me a chance to refuse, he simply hands me one of his walking poles to help with the rest of the descent. He casually calls his tent number over his shoulder as he continues onwards, so I can return the pole later. It really does attract a rare breed, this race, this sport.

The pole does help, but I've slowed dramatically by the time I reach the campsite several long hours later. My ankle's started swelling and I'm frankly exhausted. Tough to imagine how I can go through another four days of this, but I'm excited at the prospect of trying. In a bid to conserve energy for the following morning, I've decided to walk the final mile over a picturesque bridge and through a grassy field. I'm still ambling slowly as I approach the day one finish line. All competitors are cheered as they complete each day. But, seeing someone dawdling towards her, the member of the event team on the line concludes I must have been timed out at one of the checkpoints and tries to prevent me 'dibbing in' to finish. I have to persuade her that what I've actually been doing is tapering for Tuesday.

It's a terrific feeling to have completed the day. Albeit slowly – in 12 hours 41 minutes, about halfway down the field in 135th place. It's the second longest I've ever been on my feet in a race. On the plus side, I was over three hours ahead of the 11pm deadline and this was the day with the most climbing. On the minus side, every other day still has plenty of climbing, and there are four of them. And my ankle hurts.

But for now, all I care about is food and sleep. I return the pole to its kindly owner and set about finding my tent. It's a thrill to see Jez is one of my tent-mates for the week, a friendly face – not that I've found any other kind so far. We're sharing a tent with three others, and they all finished several hours ahead of me. Jez is lying fifth overall, and has been lounging about in the campsite for fully four hours by the time I stagger in. The tents have all been erected for us, but there's still plenty to do. Change out of sweaty, wet kit; eat; dispose of the day's litter; blow up sleeping mats; prepare kit and hill food for the following day; fill water bottles; and try to grab as much sleep as possible. All in the rather cramped confines of a tent. But everybody's determined to help each other and the atmosphere is highly convivial. A happy band of runners. As for Jez, I discover it was through running that he met his more usual overnight companion, his wife Gemma.

In 2009 I competed for England in the Commonwealth 100km Championships held in the pretty surroundings of Thirlmere near Keswick in the Lake District. Whilst road running is not necessarily where my heart lies, the opportunity to run for England in an international competition is a great privilege, particularly on home soil. The 100km on the road is also a distance you can really attack, usually flat and relatively fast, it's all out against the clock and there is something quite appealing about taking away some of the variables of trail running which inevitably slow you down. It turned out to be a pivotal life moment, but bizarrely not because of the gold I secured very late in the race, ahead of a good friend of mine.

It was during the post-race celebrations held in a Keswick pub that I got chatting to Sam Densen, the partner of one of my England team-mates. Fuelled by more than a few beers, I started pouring my heart out about my poor luck in finding a like-minded soulmate to share my running – and life – journey with. That conversation sowed a seed in Sam's mind, and soon I was being persuaded to consider a blind date with a running friend of hers from Dorset.

Roll forward two weeks and I was nervously waiting for Gemma to arrive in a Wiltshire lay-by. I lived in Warwick at the time, so we had arranged to meet 'halfway' and planned a walk on the downs. Gemma had run a 20-mile New York Marathon training run the night before, but showed no signs of tiredness – I was suitably impressed. The day involved 20-odd miles in all, including a nice pub lunch, tea and the brownies brought along by Gemma (winner), and a further trip to the pub for dinner afterwards.

We're now parents to baby Milo, and running remains an important part of our life together. We share the highs and lows of training and competing, making holidays out of races in various parts of the world. We often take it in turns to provide support for one another in races, adding a steely strength to our relationship and running performances. The community is second to none, you only have to feel the sense of spirit and togetherness at your Saturday morning parkrun, but having said all that, I would never have called myself a runner, and part of me still doesn't feel like a runner. It all feels quite surreal. Rugby was my thing. But I just fell into running from a lifestyle point of view.

Jez came to global prominence when he won the Ultra-Trail du Mont-Blanc. He's also broken records for the Ramsay Round in Scotland and running the length of New Zealand, but his proudest achievement is finishing third at the Western States 100. It's the world's oldest 100-mile trail race, starting in Squaw Valley, California, near the site of the 1960 Winter Olympics, and ending 100.2 miles later on a high school athletics track in Auburn.

Western States has history. It was the first race to offer belt buckles to finishers – bronze for completing the course in under 30 hours, silver if you're sub-24. There's also a staggering number of volunteers, almost five for every runner. The only way to acquire one of the highly coveted starting places is to complete one of a strictly limited list of races inside the qualifying time, and hope for the best in the draw. They talk about 'building up your Western States ticket' because the more times you fail to get in, the greater your chance of success in the following year's lottery. I've carelessly allowed my ticket to slip – even though I've run more ultras than ever in the most recent November to November qualifying period, I haven't run one of the specific races needed to get me in to WS100. It feels like losing a long-standing car insurance no-claims bonus for a minor prang. (Which I've also just done.) Western States is top of most ultra-runners' must-do lists. Jez, as an elite runner, gets in automatically – and can't get enough of it.

As an experience it's second to none, even though it doesn't have the TV coverage or any of the razzmatazz of the likes of UTMB. It's done in the right way, and it's got a lot of meaning and history to it. When you set foot on the Western States trail it just feels really special. To come from the UK, and to deliver, and to perform in the mountains, in the heat, at altitude, against all the local guys and actually be really competing, and running alongside Kílian Jornet[*] 65 miles into the race, that's rewarding. That's memorable. Kílian and I chatted as we ran, he's extremely friendly, we were just sharing the experience really. You don't have to say much when you're running alongside someone in any of these events,

---

[*] Kílian Jornet is quite simply the world's best mountain runner, winner of the world's biggest ultra-races, including Western States. More from him shortly.

you've immediately got this connection as you're just going through this challenging experience.

What appeals about the Dragon's Back Race is that you're running down Wales, it's a race with a purpose. It's a geographical journey. They're always the best challenges. Climbing 24 Munros in 24 hours in the Highlands is amazing, you know? And running from London to Birmingham on the canal is amazing because you're running from capital to second city. There's something that draws you along and that's what all these great off-road races have in common. That's why the UTMB's amazing, you're circumnavigating Mont Blanc, you're going through three different countries, all these cultures. And that takes some beating as a course. All the best races are like that, and those are the ones you want to do. It's not just about competing, it's about the experience and the opportunity.

Jez's first such journey was a relatively short one, and hardly unusual. In fact the Great North Run, Newcastle to South Shields, has been the first proper running journey for hundreds of thousands of runners, myself included. I ran the 13.1 miles as a newcomer to the sport in 2010, and was hooked. Jez experienced the crowds, the atmosphere, the all-encompassing greatness of the world's biggest half marathon about a decade earlier when he was 17. He enjoyed the day itself and also the training leading up to it. Then at university he was diagnosed with colitis, a lifelong inflammatory bowel condition. He had a moment of realisation that to give his body the best possible chance of staying well and avoiding big, life-changing operations, he needed to be fit and healthy. So he went to the gym, went jogging, stopped smoking and hardly drank alcohol.

That's big, you know, when you're at university. It impacts on your social groups. I also booked in for the London Marathon which I did as a fundraiser for Crohn's and Colitis UK, and it was amazing. I ran 3:18, had the best day of my life with family around. At the time I thought that would be the big running moment in my life. Little did I know it was just the start of it. Entering the community, making amazing friends, and starting to run off road and broaden my horizons.

So I banged out a marathon but also I was quite an outdoorsy guy. I loved hiking and backpacking. I was thinking: what sort of off-roady, challengy type stuff is there, linked to running but bringing in those other skills? I stumbled across this event called the Marathon of Britain, 175 miles, six days, basically across the Midlands. Take a week off work and spend it with all these crazy like-minded people! I shared that experience with those guys and I'm still in touch with a lot of them now. That was my entry into the really long stuff and it's very surreal even to this day to think that I did so well and managed to win it. I was like, I can be good at this.

'Good' doesn't really begin to cover it. I've counted 15 significant race wins in Jez Bragg's career and I've probably missed some. But I wonder whether juggling a full-time job, training, and now becoming a father has taken its toll. It can't be easy staying at the top of his game.

It's not, and it's always been a battle ever since I started really. But it's a choice I've made deliberately because I need to be challenged in other aspects of my life and career's important to me. I enjoy what I do, I'm a project manager for theatres. I've had little spells where I've put it down for three or four months and done a bit of travelling, but I've always come back to it. I know it's compromised some of my performances in the sense that I probably don't sleep and rest as much as I should do, and I'm burning the candle at both ends. Trying to keep family and friends, and job, and running career, and sponsors, all those balls in the air, it's difficult at times. But it's also very rewarding when you're pulling amazing stuff off. I think you almost get even more credibility for that, for having a relatively normal life as well as being put on a pedestal as a really good runner.

In future, now I'm a dad, I don't know whether I'm going to be racing quite so much. I've been running competitively for 14 years now, and you do have an elite running lifespan. I have to face reality a bit. Sharpness is perhaps not quite there, but I'm not beating myself up too much if I can't quite get to the level I've been at previously. I keep on trying but it's a really hard place to get to and your body has to be able to withstand it. Recovery time does slow down. I'm becoming more philosophical and I'm certainly becoming more appreciative of what I've done previously, as opposed to always looking forward.

But that's the great thing about this sport. There are always slightly different opportunities to turn to, and I think I'm heading towards one-off challenge adventures. You know, not necessarily running down New Zealand, but one of the long distance paths in the UK or a group of Munros (mountains over 3,000 feet) in Scotland. There are all these semi-underground UK records which these old boys in their plimsolls set in the 1970s and '80s which are just crying out for me to have a crack at. Something that's not quite so obvious to people but would still be an amazing adventure – it motivates me and gets me out on the wild hills.

Hills don't get much wilder than day one of the Dragon's Back Race though, do they? I revisit our conversation from the previous month when I asked Jez to rate the slopes above Conwy on a wilderness score out of 10, and was disappointed when he said six. 'Now I know what you meant, Jez,' I say with an indecent amount of knowing pride. 'Some of that terrain between Tryfan and Snowdon, that's 10, right? Crib Goch – I mean, of course!'

Some of the others sharing our tent perk up at this point. Ed, Dave and Huw (who'd later describe the race as 'harder than passing a kidney stone and then trying to put it back') raise a collective eyebrow. Day one, I learn, had the most climbing, but only just. Day two, they tell me gleefully, day two will have the wildest terrain.

'Just you wait until you reach the Rhinogydd. That's 10.'

Oh shit.

6. machynlleth

Not much sleep, four hours if I'm lucky. I'm keen to set off as early as possible to give myself the greatest possible chance of finishing day two. A multi-day ultra is a balancing act, I'm learning. More rest to help you recover from the previous day, or more time in the mountains to help you complete today? I opt for option B, and get up (as quietly as possible because everyone else in the tent is still sleeping) at 4:45am. Lots to do before the earliest official departure time of 6am.

Not least, attend to my burgeoning blister collection. My feet are rubbed raw in several places, but I hadn't really paid attention to the pain yesterday as I was so worried about the ankle. Only thing to do this morning is borrow some tape, cover them all up, hope for the best.

Next, food – breakfast – which opens at 5. The whole week's campsite catering is vegetarian, and it's all fantastic. This morning's fare includes cereal, lots of it, eggs on toast, veggie sausages, more cereal, and a gallon of milky coffee. I bolt down as much as I can, but with one eye on the watch – time is ticking towards 6am and I still have loads to do before setting off. Wash up my plastic plate, bowl, camping cutlery and mug and repack them in the large dry bag along with the sleeping bag, mat and camp clothes. That'll be transported to tonight's campsite. After that, the smaller dry bag needs restocking with stuff I might need at the drop point: extra food, blister plasters, painkillers, dry clothes. Then it's the running rucksack which I'll carry with me all day – water, food, phone and a big long list of mandatory equipment: survival bag, map and compass, headtorch with spare batteries, whistle, spare warm top, hat, gloves, waterproof jacket (with taped seams and a hood), waterproof trousers (with taped seams), money (at least £50 in case of emergency taxi) and a waterproof pencil or chinagraph. There's a spot check before the start of each day and you never know what they're going to ask to see. I consider risking it and dispensing with the cheap, bulky survival blanket I ordered online – but lose my nerve and pack it reluctantly. Good thing too, as the blanket is one of the two random items I'm asked to show (the compass is the other).

In amongst all the personal admin, I managed to find someone with the same Garmin as me, and I return his charging lead to his tent along with his watch, which I've charged from my power pack. A quick check of the noticeboard for last-minute route alterations, then squelch back into the mountain running shoes, Inov-8 Roclites, which are still soaking wet from yesterday. The early morning dew hasn't helped. This isn't as bad as it sounds – I know both feet will be sodden soon enough, so best get it over with early. And I actually find I don't much mind having wet feet all day.

Finally, at almost half past 6, I'm ready to leave. The day begins with a long climb up Cnicht. It's not an especially tall mountain but this is my first experience of climbing in thick fog – or 'heavy clag' as the veterans would call it. Visibility is down to a few metres and the going is tough. The earliest starters are half an hour ahead of me up the mountainside, while the more competitive runners have yet to set off, doubtless waiting for the clag to clear. I find myself properly alone for the first time in the race. And because of the poor visibility, I do feel the solitude.

As I climb, a chance to reflect. To be sure, I wasn't prepared for this, but I'm absolutely loving the challenge. There are no aid stations, nobody to give you a cake and a cuddle every few miles. There are few paths or pre-marked routes. It's just you, a map and the mountains. You look around at the vast expanse of Snowdonia – and it's all yours. This is the difference between a mountain race and a trail race. Here you get to choose the route – go any way you like, just get to all the checkpoints and reach the cut-offs on time.

I go wrong coming down from Cnicht and end up some way off course. I first suspect I've made a mistake when I hear distant voices, carried on the wind, from somewhere far to my right. Surely these are fellow Dragon's Back runners; who else would be out on top of a mountain so early on a morning like this? I have a moment of panic. I check the watch but it's being weird. So I'm alone in the clag, lost in the mountains, with almost no visibility and an increasingly torturous ankle. Suddenly I'm not enjoying this much any more.

But then, I think, that's the point of this race. The dragon statues they give out at the finish wouldn't be so coveted if they were easy to earn. You just need to be... *competent* in a situation like this. I reach for a caffeinated gel in a bid to defibrillate myself. Then I run towards the voices, scouring the map and my surroundings for a clue about my position. If in doubt, I learned yesterday, head upwards. They don't miss many opportunities to put those checkpoint boxes on peaks.

Mercifully the clag clears. I take stock, realise where I've gone wrong (I'd almost doubled back on myself) and set out to put it right. Aiming for another summit, then a reservoir in the valley below, a third summit – it's suddenly so much easier now I can see.

The visibility comes and goes, as does my mojo. A gloriously runnable stretch of short grass, and my spirits soar. An ill-judged descent resulting in my upper arm being torn by barbed wire, and the mojo dies off again. I realise to my horror that I'm struggling to make the 3pm cut-off time at the drop bag point.

Negative thoughts and emotions course through me, threatening to drown out everything else. I consider calling my wife but fear I might cry. My ankle is in bits, a metaphor for my mind.

I take another wrong turn and end up wading down a steep bank of knee-deep heather when I could have been running on an actual path. The three people I overtook whilst I was feeling positive all go back past me. Two of them are running non-competitively as they were timed out yesterday. It's much less of a big deal for them whether they make the 3pm deadline. Which, it seems, I almost certainly won't. I step into what looks a tiny puddle and disappear up to my waist. I almost lose a shoe trying to haul myself up. I thought this sort of thing only happened in cartoons.

Checkpoint 4 crosses a railway line and the suggested latest arrival time is 11am. Good job these checkpoints don't have cut-offs or I'd have missed it by a long way: it's almost afternoon. I've been losing time ever since I started and it's clear which way my race is heading. The negativity is tough to turn off. I definitely won't make the 3pm drop bag cut-off; what's the point in even trying?

Now I do phone my wife. She answers, bright and enthusiastic, asks me how it's going, and something akin to grief comes crashing down over me. I'm tired, hurting, bleeding, way out of my depth, I tell her through barely concealed sobs. I'm also furious with myself for calling Caroline in the midst of my misery. Because this pain is self-inflicted. Nobody's forcing me to be here.

'Stay right where you are,' says Caroline. 'And don't move!'

'What?'

'Stay where you are. I'm coming to get you.'

'Caroline, you're a six-hour drive away in London. We have kids who need picking up from school and nursery. Thank you but obviously, no thank you.'

'I'll sort all that on the way. Just stay where you are.'

What I needed – and expected – to hear was *Stop feeling sorry for yourself and get on with it*. But this works just as well. I thank Caroline, apologise for pouring self-pity down the line at her, and take stock. What an amazing, loving wife I have; I'm beyond lucky.

All those negative emotions swirling around are difficult to tame once they've started running wild. But in amongst them all, a flicker of positive thought to hang on to and build on.

I've never had a DNF (Did Not Finish) next to my name in any race I've ever run. However badly things have turned, however tempted I've sometimes been to pull out, I've always found the will to finish. A little voice in the back of my mind reminds me of that. If I'm going to miss the cut-off and be disqualified, I'm going to go down fighting.

I stop grappling with the agony in my ankle. You can be in pain without suffering. Radical acceptance they call it, and it's enormously freeing. This doesn't just hold true in an ultra. Life in general is better when you focus on the good stuff. I once read somewhere that 'the quality of an experience is directly related to the quality of your thoughts'. I like that. Catch the negative emotions before they take control and hang on to something positive like gratitude.

Or community. As we run through a village and up a steep road, I see a competitor heading towards me from the opposite direction. A huge smile emerges from the middle of his beard as we meet by a crossing and I turn right while he goes left. He's an American called Ricky and has vast experience of orienteering. He even runs his own adventure company. Out in the wild mountains where map reading is tricky, there's nobody better. But on this rare road section, Ricky got sloppy, overconfident, and missed a turning. He's just added an unnecessary 10km to his journey and the extra hour will probably make the difference between reaching the cut-off on time – and not. But still, Ricky's smiling. He's just happy to be here. And I'm thrilled to have met him.

The lesson I learned after my embarrassing phone call home is reinforced in concrete.

For the next few hours, Ricky and I team up. There's no talk of giving up and taking it easy. This is an all-out assault on our 3pm deadline, and despite the pain, discomfort, stress – it feels fantastic. We make it with 20 minutes to go.

More positive energy comes my way in the shape of a happy, wise-cracking volunteer called Stuart. Somehow, in the rush to get here, I've lost my map. Must've dropped it somewhere in the woods or mountains. (To be honest, despite his missed turning fiasco, Ricky's skills with a map are far superior to mine and I've basically been following him.) Stuart conjures a new map from nowhere, then proceeds to find some fresh tape. The blisters on my feet and heels have become craters, and there are six of them of varying depths.

I have exactly 20 minutes before I have to hand back my drop bag and get going again, and take 19 of them. Stuart's with me throughout, helping, making jokes, generally being brilliant. I tell him I owe him a beer (which I still do to this day – a fact he frequently emails to remind me).

At one minute to three I set off into the Rhinogydd. I miss the commotion at a minute *past* three, when a competitor arrives just after the cut-off and is told he can't continue. He'd been flying, one of the quicker runners on day one, but simply set off too late today and compounded the error by treating himself to a pit stop in a pub in the inviting village of Maentwrog. He's furious about it, but rules are rules.

Meanwhile I have eight hours to make it to camp. I don't really fancy my chances, but I'm definitely going to give it my very best shot. A long climb, several false summits, some staggering views in the sunshine, then a truly ridiculous descent. A sheer slope covered in mammoth boulders and heather. I step down from one huge rock onto another covered in heather. My foot finds air. As I'm falling there's a moment when I fear the worst. A split second later and I land on solid ground, chest deep in boulders. *This is finally it*, I think. *This is 10 out of 10 on Jez's wild terrain scale.*

It's also 10 out of 10 on the beauty scale, and 11 out of 10 on the remoteness scale. There's nobody else for miles and miles around. The only other humans up here are Dragon's Back competitors struggling over boulders, puffing up never-ending mountainsides, hoping to reach the distant campsite before 11 pm.

On the way up to each mountain top are at least half a dozen false summits. Every descent is hard, technical, ankle-obliterating. It's agonisingly slow-going. Eventually the final summit is slain, the final descent negotiated.

Just one last twist with the campsite in sight: a two-mile detour through a darkening wood and up a sharp slope. I suspect it's the organisers' idea of humour, and so it proves. Shane Ohly, race director, and Gary Tompsett, in charge of the course, love nothing better than leaving an unwelcome surprise for exhausted competitors. This is what my late granny would have called a Japanese ambush. During the Second World War, the Japanese would wait until American patrols were almost back at base, and starting to relax, before attacking. It's the modern-day, Welsh mountain version of the Japanese ambush that basically does for me.

The final half-mile to camp is on a road down a gentle hill. On a good day, less than three minutes. Even at the end of an ultra, no more than five or six. But suddenly, towards the end of that extra section in those trees, my ankle decides it's had enough.

I'm usually pretty good at disassociating myself from pain. But however hard I try now, I fail. That final half mile takes 20 minutes to hobble. I'm completely broken. The Welsh mountains have chewed me up and spat me out.

I'm inside the cut-off when I dib in to end the day, but not by much. My tent-mates are already sleeping. I crave sleep, but have to get sorted first. I'm freezing, dizzy with hunger, utterly dehydrated. But my priority is my ankle, so I head to the medical tent. I'm not expecting much sympathy and I'm not disappointed.

'You're the guy who had an ankle sprain before he started, aren't you?'

'Er, yes.'

'Who wouldn't listen to medical advice and said you were going to run regardless?'

'Yes. Sorry about that. My bad. But is there anything you can do, please?'

'Of course. Don't worry. I can fix that for you now.'

I breathe a huge sigh of relief as the doctor starts to rummage in her white coat for something, tape presumably, to sort out my ankle. What emerges in her hand is a magic wand. An actual black plastic stick with white ends. She waves it in the direction of my ankle.

'There you go. All sorted.'

Hilarious.

Fair enough, though. And what did I expect? I'm told to report back the following morning.

The sleeping tents are frustratingly far away from where food's being served, and ours is at the very far end of the campsite. It's the sort of thing you only notice when you're injured. So a long limp to collect plate and cutlery, and a long limp back to eat. I'm shivering, and somebody lends me a coat.

There are showers here, proper showers, the only ones we'll see all week. The idea of standing under warm water and getting clean is ridiculously appealing. But the showers are in a separate block a further quarter of a mile away. No chance. I'm so tired, and hurting so much, that I try to minimise the admin. Forget washing up, brushing teeth, even cleaning my face, hands and the blood off my arm. Forget the toilets, which again I decide are too far away. I wee behind a tree.

I stumble into the tent, and blunder about in the dark whilst trying to be as quiet as possible so as not to wake anyone. Finding a dry top to wear, blowing up the mat, climbing into the sleeping bag – I must wake everyone but they're all kind enough to pretend to slumber on. It's half past midnight by the time I set the alarm for half past four.

The following morning sees precious little improvement from the ankle. I can't see how on earth I'm going to get through today, but try to banish the negative thoughts. I'll just do what I can. I know the ankle is damaged, but hope that somehow the pain recedes enough for me to be able to run on it again. You never know, perhaps a good hard climb is exactly what it needs. Even inside my head, the optimism sounds hollow.

Back to the medical tent for some strapping. They do what they can for the ankle, then take a look at my blisters and inform me that they're similarly beyond help. But they kindly dress them anyway to minimise the pain. I'm ravenously hungry, despite only eating a few hours ago, and hobble back to the tent for my plate. It takes me a long time to get sorted enough to leave.

Out of the campsite, through the market town of Dolgellau and up a long path next to a charming waterfall. I make sure I enjoy these moments, as I'm not sure how many more there'll be. A farmer waits by a gate and offers sweets, encouragement and cups of water. A cow with a calf starts at me in a field; I didn't even know cows did that. Then, heart racing, over a stile and back into the mountains for the final push through Snowdonia.

The climb to the top of Gau Graig takes an awful lot longer than it should. Whatever I try I can't shake off the permanent ankle pain – or prevent it slowing me down. It's extremely frustrating. I keep hoping the hurt will simply evaporate. I'm limping. My pace is passive, plodding, ponderous.

So it comes as a bit of a shock when I catch someone up. It seems he's suffering more than I am, with a suspected broken bone in the bottom of his foot. He winces every time he puts any weight on it. His race is clearly run but the trouble is, he's miles from anywhere on top of a Welsh mountain in thick clag.

We hobble on together, towards the next checkpoint on top of Cadair Idris, the most famous peak in southern Snowdonia and one of the most popular for walkers and hikers. The views from the top are said to be spectacular, even by the lofty standards of the past few days. Mountainscapes are health food for the soul.

Not today. The visibility is so poor, we have to be careful not to blunder onto any cliff edge. It's said that anyone who sleeps on the slopes of Cadair Idris will awaken the following morning a madman or a poet. The pace we're travelling, spending the night up here is a proper possibility.

Eventually we make it to the summit, and make three unexpected new friends. One of them is simply thrilled to be up there and doesn't give two hoots about the lack of a view. He's called Sherlock, and he is scampering and sniffing around delightedly. His tail's wagging so hard, it might just fan away all the fog. Sherlock the Beagle, I later learn, is famous in mountain racing circles. Indeed he has more

Instagram followers than his owners, Jen and Marcus Scotney. At almost exactly the same time as I'm meeting his dog, Marcus takes the race lead from the 2015 winner, Jim Mann, and it's a lead he won't relinquish. (Jim, to general astonishment, makes a massive navigational error, adding an extra hour and 15 minutes to his race.) Jen's up there too, looking almost as content as her dog. She's wearing a big, happy smile and holding a camera. We're just telling her about Mark's injury issue when another man appears, almost miraculously, out of the fog. He's from mountain rescue, off duty, choosing to spend his free Wednesday morning climbing a mountain in bad weather. He offers to nurse my new friend back down to his car, then drive him somewhere useful.

'I'd better get a wiggle on,' I say to Sherlock and Jen, and stumble onwards. I'm thinking perhaps it's a day for miracles. First the appearance of the mountain rescue bloke. Next, if possible, some kind of spectacular improvement in my ankle. No sign of it yet, mind.

The following four hours are both excruciating and wonderful. I realise at one point that I'm on top of a mountain in fog, in pain, injured, with no battery in my GPS watch and as far as I know, miles from the nearest person. If you'd presented me with that situation a week previously, I'd have confidently told you that I'd be panicking. And yet I'm not. I'm actually quite content.

Three days in the Welsh mountains, and I seem to have learned some competence. The pain is what it is, nothing I can do about it. I have a map and two working legs – and I'm certain I'll be fine. It's a rather agreeable sensation. I press onwards towards Machynlleth and its famous clock tower. I know I'll get there eventually. Whether I'll be at the designated drop point car park before the 16:30 cut-off time is debatable.

Soon debatable becomes unlikely. And before long, unlikely becomes impossible. Ironically this realisation dawns when I'm on a fantastically runnable, grassy footpath winding its way gently downhill through a field. It's the sort of path I'm used to, the sort of terrain I've trained on – and actually the sort of thing there'll be a lot more of now the race has left Snowdonia. But I won't see any of that. The remote and rarely visited hills of the Elan Valley of day four, the Cambrian Mountains and Brecon Beacons of day five – those will be for others to enjoy.

Just as I'm beginning to feel guilty about how long they'll have to wait for me at the drop bag point – and wondering whether to call to tell them not to bother, that I'll get a cab to the campsite – I hear two people tearing downhill behind me, chatting as they go. I turn to see two experienced trail runners galloping over the grass at ridiculous speed, yet making it all seem effortless. I move across to let them pass but I'm surprised when they screech to a halt beside me.

These are the guys who run the course before and behind us, setting up the checkpoint boxes 24 hours before the competitors get to them, and clearing up after we've gone through. There are several such teams working in tandem.

'Hi mate. We've got a van parked at the bottom of this hill. We'll give you a lift to Machynlleth.'

The offer does sound tempting, and my ankle could certainly do with the rest. However, there's no way I'm pulling out before I need to. I've never failed to finish a race, any race. It's not yet cut-off time so technically, I'm still in this.

'Technically,' I tell them, 'I'm still in this. It's not yet half past four. Thank you, but no thank you.'

'Suit yourself,' they say. 'Only thing is, it will be half past four soon, after which you'll have another two mountains to climb on that ankle.'

They walk with me whilst I dither. When we reach the van, I pause, then with a heavy heart I open the passenger door. My race is run.

It's not the injured ankle that stops me finishing the Dragon's Back Race, though it certainly doesn't help. This is the toughest multi-stage race in the world; those who complete it are awesome. Who am I to think that with minimal mountain training I could be a match for any of them? Put simply, my best shot hasn't been good enough.

There's a 'leave me alone and don't speak to me' area in the drop bag point. I'm disappointed to see several familiar faces already there: Ricky the smiling American from yesterday; Chris who I first met during a 100-miler in the South Downs the previous summer; and of course my friend with his damaged heel. As you can imagine, the mood is sombre.

7. london

On the plus side, it means I reach the campsite early enough to meet some of the leading runners. On previous days they've been safely tucked up in bed by the time I've staggered into the finish. Over dinner I tell Marcus Scotney how I've fallen in love with his dog.

'I hope you're following him on Instagram?'

'Yes, I... Hang on. What? No I don't have Instagram. But your dog does?'

'Sherlockthebeagle1. He's got more than twice the followers I have. Thousands of them. Which is a fair amount. For a beagle.'

It is, I agree. And doubly impressive to have more followers than your owner, when your owner has several spheres to pick from. Marcus isn't only an elite mountain runner. He's also an actor, a sports therapist and a coach. As well as a husband and father. So what made him decide to put the rest of his life on hold and take on the Dragon's Back Race?

I've been involved in the long-distance running scene for years. And these stories about the original race, they are just out there. You know, it was talked about. This one-off event which took place in 1992. And it was just mythical. It's always been such an iconic event, which was only held once.

And then in 2012, I worked with Shane Ohly when he decided to re-introduce it. And I was just in awe of the likes of Steve Birkinshaw, who won it, interviewing him, and seeing him run. Just absolutely phenomenal. And I just thought it was way beyond me. You know, this kind of running like that. The five days, over that kind of terrain. Also watching Helene Diamantides, winner of the original race, come back again.

Then I got talked into doing Cape Wrath*, which seemed a lot more my type of running. It's more trail, less mountainous. But it's a lot more remote than the Dragon's Back. If you think Wales is remote, Cape Wrath is completely out there. You don't see anybody all day, other than your fellow competitors. No drop bags to pick up. Just wild.

I surprised myself by winning Cape Wrath. Didn't know how my body was going to cope with multi-stage races, being so small and lightweight. I always thought it needs to be a lot more bigger, a bit more bulk, to just burn off. But when I came back from Cape Wrath, I was like, oh, I've got to do more of these. And no other race came anywhere near to the profile or the toughness of Cape Wrath, other than the Dragon's Back. And I just thought, well let's give it a try.

What also draws me to these things is the journey. A lot of races go in a circle, start and finish at the same place. But here there's such a linear journey. And you're in such wilderness, where you just don't normally go and run. And it's not just a one-off race. You've got to do it day in, day out, which becomes a bit of a holiday as well. It sounds weird, but it's a way of looking at it. Because for five days you're literally just switched off from the world. No phone, tweets, email, or anything like that. So there's a real sense that you are isolated and just immersed in the event.

Three days gone in Wales, and just like the previous year in the Highlands of Scotland, Marcus has surprised himself by how well he's fared. He took the lead today, but didn't know about it until just before he came into camp. Jim Mann, defending champion, pre-race favourite, leader after two days, made a big navigational error and it cost him. He

---

* Ourea Events, who stage the Dragon's Back Race every two years, also put on the biennial Cape Wrath Ultra in even-numbered years. It's an eight-day expedition weaving 400km through the Highlands of Scotland. Longer than its Welsh sister, more remote, perhaps even more beautiful. But easier.

came off Cadair Idris on the wrong ridge, and took a long time to figure out his mistake. He'd started late and suddenly found himself under pressure to make the cut-off, the same one I'd missed, at the support point in Machynlleth. Very quickly it became survival mode. Being Jim Mann, he made the cut-off comfortably in the end. But he lost a ton of time and the lead.

The next time I speak to Marcus, it's a few weeks after he managed to keep Jim at bay for two days and hang on for a memorable victory. He hadn't seemed it when we were chatting over dinner in the campsite, but he was feeling stressed. Now he had a lead to protect.

Thursday was the day I was most worried about. I made two really silly navigation errors. First I made a mistake going to Checkpoint 1. I should have researched Jim's line. Jim took a much shorter line and I lost about 15 minutes. And then Checkpoint 4, I overshot by a few minutes, because I saw a cameraman on the hill and just legged it to him. I wasn't focusing on my navigation, like an idiot. Kind of a headless chicken. And then I had to turn around and run back, and go past a couple of other competitors, which was quite embarrassing. But in some ways it adds to the adrenaline. You're like, right, this is proper racing. This is one of the reasons you do it. And you're just trying to fight to survive, and you don't know how Jim's doing, or what other people are doing. You get tired and fatigued, but you're trying to maintain a fast pace without breaking yourself down. It was so hot. And I was struggling with my knee as well.

I wondered if there was a precise point he would have stopped, even whilst leading the Dragon's Back Race, because his knee was too sore. When he couldn't run any more? Or would he have pushed on regardless? When Goran Ivanišević reached his first Wimbledon final, he was struggling with an injury. Asked if he might pull out, he said, 'It's the final of Wimbledon. Even if I'm dead, I'll play.' So just how 'Goran' is Marcus? How 'Goran' are any of us?

Yeah. I mean this is always interesting. Because there's a real element of the psychological. A part where, as you probably discovered, *I just hurt*. Whatever you're doing, you get to a point and your body just hurts. It naturally hurts. You're trying to switch off that hurt, ignore it as best you can, knowing that everybody else is hurting. As long as I can continue to move at a reasonable-ish pace, then I know I'm OK. When things are really swelling up, that's when I worry.

And that's what happened when I got to the camp on the Thursday night. I stopped running, and the knee suddenly swelled up, and I lost a lot of movement in it. I was really hobbling around and struggling to walk. That's when alarm bells are starting to ring. Something's gone wrong here. Something's not quite right. But a lot can happen in 12 hours – sleeping, and resting. And initially I was just thinking, right, well, let's just run with Jim on Friday. You know, let's just run in together. We've had a good battle. And just the opportunity to finish the race could be a good result. And a thing which I never thought I could do anyway.

But I sat in the river, did self-acupuncture on my leg. A lot of icing. And then woke up Friday morning and I just thought, stuff this: I've come this far, it's only another 33 miles, final day – let's just see what can happen, really. I felt so much better on the last morning. I taped up the knee. And I was just like, what's the worst that can happen? I can injure myself and be off for six weeks. But then there's the opportunity of winning the Berghaus Dragon's Back Race.

Marcus had an eight-minute lead over Jim. Just eight minutes separated the top two contenders after over 30 hours of racing. The organisers persuaded them to stagger their start times on Friday so Jim would be chasing Marcus down. Whoever crossed the finishing line first would win.

I went out, and I ran scared that whole morning. I was literally looking over my shoulder every five minutes, expecting Jim to come charging me down. I knew he knew all the little shortcuts and little trods to take. It's proper racing, and the chasing start made it really exciting, even for people at home dot watching*.

I fell over so many times. It was just hilarious. Because obviously my legs weren't quite working right. And I was pushing myself. I kept expecting him to pop up behind me. The whole way, across the Black Mountain and over on the Brecon Beacons, I just expected him to pop up behind me. And every time I could see a runner in the distance, or anybody in the distance, I'd think, that's Jim. He's coming. He's charging me down.

Ian Corless was up in the mountain again taking photographs. I asked him if he knew where Jim was, and he said no, he had no idea where anybody was.

So it wasn't until the castle, when we got down off the Brecon Beacons, when I thought, this is in the bag now. I knew once I hit tarmac, got into road-running mode, I could probably keep Jim off. Even if he closed me down, I could take 30 seconds out of him going downhill. It was in the bag.

It's really hard to kind of summarise how that felt. It was such a sense of relief and an emotional drain. Because you've literally just pushed yourself so hard, and so far beyond what you're normally capable of doing. It took a couple of days for it all to sink in, that I'd actually won it. And initially, I just wanted to lie down. Rest my leg. As soon as I stopped it just gave way. The body shut down. It was like, that's it. We're done. Don't expect us to work any more.

Like when I walked back to the car and Jen took a short video, which she posted on Twitter, of me trying to walk towards it. And I'm just completely peg-legged, can hardly move at all. It's like the body knows

---

* All competitors had GPS trackers. It's surprisingly engaging watching a small numbered dot travel ever so slowly across the Welsh countryside. My wife says she knew I'd had it when my dot started moving much slower than all the other dots.

exactly how far to push it. You cross the line and that's it, the body just goes shoonk, shuts straight down. Everybody kept asking, 'Do you want a chair?' And I was like, 'No, I need to lie down.'

And afterwards it was amazing. That weird, mixed emotion. To be reunited with Jen, and to know that I'd achieved something which I had always thought was way beyond me. And to win it quite emphatically, as I did, to set a new course record, to break 38 hours... yeah, at times it's still sinking in. Now, when I'm out training, I find myself reminiscing. It's quite a good motivator.

But training for what? After winning the Cape Wrath Ultra and Dragon's Back Race back to back, where do you go from there? In Marcus's case, Costa Rica. The notorious Coastal Challenge. A six-day, 146-mile trek through jungle, along beaches, over mountains and across rivers. The major problem? Searing heat and 95% humidity. I once practically passed out after a 40-minute jungle jog on the Thailand-Myanmar border. I hesitate to mention it to Marcus, but red-heads don't tend to do too well in ridiculously hot and humid conditions.

Yeah, I didn't used to be any good in the heat at all. But a couple of summers ago I embraced it. And now I love it. I'm going to get into a heat chamber a couple of times, just to get used to it. Again, it's partly mental. If you say, I don't like heat, or I can't cope with hills, or rain, or wind, anything like that, then it becomes a hurdle that will stop you. But if you decide yes, I can cope with it, then you find you can and do. During the heat on the fourth day of the Dragon's Back, I was like, yeah, I love this. Bring it on.

Since then I've also realised I can do gnarly and hard. I've just been watching the Tor des Géants, and that looks pretty bonkers. But there's so much choice. It's unbelievable really. I'm quite drawn to some of the big events too, the big 100-milers like Western States. Oh, and Barkley.

The trouble with this sport, I've found, with the speed it's growing, is that your list just can't keep up. Both Tor des Géants and Barkley are on mine, albeit quite low down the realistic list and high on the aspirational, if-I-ever-get-good-enough list. I heard about Tor des Géants from GB ultra-runner Debbie Martin-Consani (from whom more later) whilst she was crewing for her husband Marco, a fellow international, in the Spartathlon.

TDG sounds amazing, but it almost broke her. And that, with Debbie, is saying something. Run every September in Courmayeur, it follows the Alta Via 1 and Alta Via 2 around the Valle d'Aosta, 200 miles with an altitude range of 80,000 feet. Competitors decide when and where to rest. The race starts on Sunday morning and you've got until the following Saturday afternoon to complete it. Sounds easy. Really and truly – because of the climbing – isn't.

A little like the Barkley Marathons. A 60-hour time limit to run five loops of around 20 miles each. That's just four marathons averaging 15 hours each. Most 100-mile races have a 30-hour cut-off, and people can generally walk much of the way and still get their belt buckle. And yet. The Barkley Marathons, brainchild of the legendary Lazarus Lake (not his real name), can justifiably and uncontroversially be described as the toughest ultra in the world. It has a 1% success rate. That's 1%. Only 15 runners have ever completed the race; most years nobody finishes.

There's climbing you see. Lots of climbing. Some 5km vertical ascent every loop, and it's not on footpaths, it's in wild mountains. You're basically bushwhacking. Oh and the quirks. You give Lazarus (his real name is Gary Cantrell) a number plate from your car as the entry fee. Unless you've previously completed the race, if you're one of those 15 people, in which case you give him a packet of Camel Lights. But even to enter in the first place, that's a conundrum in itself.

You've got to send an email, at midnight on Christmas Day, with an essay about why you deserve a place. That's midnight in Laz's time zone, but you have to guess which one that is. If you're early or late, you're out. Sometimes you hear back right away (successful applicants get a 'commiserations' email), sometimes not for ages. It messes with your head, even before you begin. Eventually you'll be told the race venue and date.

Then one night you'll find yourself lying in a tent in the Cumberland Mountains of Eastern Tennessee, half asleep, along with 34 other nervous runners, and some time between 11pm and 11am you'll hear a conch shell being blown. Then you'll know you're 60 minutes from the start. From almost certain doom. A few hours previously, you'll have been shown a course map (it changes every year) that you can copy onto a map you've purchased. Phones, watches and GPS equipment are all banned. The printed set of course directions are notoriously difficult to follow, even with a compass. One competitor famously became so hopelessly lost that he ended up wandering for a day and a half in a different county. It emerged that in 32 hours, he'd managed to cover just two miles of the actual course. Which is meant to be 100 miles but it's said to be as long as 130.

The race begins when Lazarus lights a cigarette, and tradition dictates that you don't let him see you run. So you all walk briskly until you're out of sight, then embark on running's version of *Mission Impossible*. To prove you haven't cut the course, you have to find several books along the route and rip out the page corresponding to your race number. If you're wearing '1', then you're the annual 'sacrificial virgin', the person deemed least likely to complete a single lap.

Throughout the first night, the sound of a bugle rings out over the mountainside. It's Laz playing 'The Last Post' whenever anyone drops out. Most do on the first loop; almost everyone does eventually. In 2017, a Canadian competitor missed the 60-hour deadline by six seconds.

If you do finish (which you won't), you reach a yellow gate and push a button saying 'That was easy'.

The Barkley Marathons, Tor des Géants, Western States 100, Coastal Challenge... it seems elite mountain runners like Marcus have never-ending lists like the rest of us. But just how much of Marcus Scotney is a professional athlete and how much is a professional actor?

That's a good question. To be honest I wish I was more professional actor than professional runner. I also do sports therapy and coaching on the side. I'm probably 40% professional runner. And then, 30% actor first, and 30% coach and therapist.

When leaving for something like the Dragon's Back, I make sure I just focus on the running, and tell my agent that I'm not available for acting work that week. I control my own clinic diary. And the coaching I do mobile anyway, all online. It's like juggling really, and these days quite a few professional runners do it that way.

Also I'm just fortunate where I live in the Peak District that I can train really easily, on rough ground as well, which makes a big difference.

A major victory like the Dragon's Back has opened up many more opportunities for Marcus. Costa Rica came off the back of it. But unlike big city marathons, there's little money in being invited to race the iconic events.

I wish! No, I only get a small amount of financial support from Hoka. So when I say I'm a pro runner, it means I get a tiny amount stipend and all my kit is supplied. And I get travel expenses covered and the opportunities to go away and race. So, yes, winning Dragon's Back means more opportunities and more press coverage, which means I get more coaching clients, more coaching work. It just raises your profile.

It's really been interesting. Going back to the late 1990s, ultra-running was such a tiny, tiny scene. We didn't have ultras, just a few long-distance races. And it's really interesting watching how the scene has completely grown from this tiny little niche sport into this huge kind of machine. This monstrosity.

And it's partly fuelled by social media, which is such a big driver. We didn't have social media then so people didn't know about races. When Mark Hartell did his 24-hour Lakeland Round* it wasn't recorded.

---

* In 1997 an IT professional from Stoke climbed 77 of the Lake District's highest peaks in a single day. The record is considered unbreakable.

Whereas now people are becoming professional athletes because of social media.

I discover how right he is about social media on the train home from Wales. The organisers give us a lift to Aberystwyth station, us race dropouts, and I begin the torturous, four-train journey home. By now the ankle has swollen to the approximate size of a watermelon. It looks like my leg has been fitted upside down. Every time I change trains, it's a pantomime ordeal. Once I have to go up and over a bridge to change platforms. But I'm moving so agonisingly slowly that I can only watch my next train arrive, open and close its doors, and depart – whilst I limp ineffectually towards it. It's a two-hour wait for the next one.

However, with time on my side and the luxury of phone reception, I turn on Twitter to find an unprecedented number of messages. Literally thousands and thousands of them, congratulatory in tone for two-and-a-half days, then commiserating. Some aren't even meant for me, but I've been tagged into conversations that have gone on for days. I'm startled by how many people have been following the race on Twitter, Facebook, Instagram…. We get some of the biggest pop stars in the world visiting Radio 2, yet the sheer intensity of social media traffic for a niche race in Wales seems almost comparable. Though perhaps that's an over-reaction from somebody who's been blissfully off the grid for four days.

I finally arrive back at Euston and the bustle and business of rush hour jars disturbingly. Twenty-four hours ago I was alone in clag on top of a deserted mountain, limping contentedly. Now I'm moving even slower through a crowded railway station. The commuters have no pity or patience for the hobbling man carrying two large bags on his shoulders. I'm jostled and tutted at. Welcome home.

8. corinth

Back in Greece, and I'm still fretting about running too fast. Through the ancient city of Corinth, past the famous ruins, 50 miles and a third of the race gone, and suddenly we're off the busy main road and onto dirt tracks through olive groves and open countryside. The change is very welcome.

The road meanders upwards for the first significant climb of the Spartathlon. I've yet to slow to a hike for any gradient, but I'm currently running with an amiable, Boston-based Irishman called Padraig and it doesn't take much mutual persuading for us both to give our quads a bit of a rest.

'Should we perhaps walk...?'

'Yes, let's definitely walk this hill.'

Apparently the man who came fourth last year walked every single uphill, however short or mild. The course is gently undulating throughout, so it beggars belief how quickly he must have run the flats and downhills if that's true. The thought also occurs that he'd have probably finished higher than fourth if he'd run some hills. With a few notable exceptions, the hills are really very 'runnable'.

This is one of the exceptions. The slope is longer and steeper than it looks so we have time to chat and swap stories. Padraig tells me about a blatant episode of cheating he recently encountered in a 100-mile race in the USA. On a course he knows well, he approached a left turn at a T-junction only to see a fellow competitor go straight across in front of him, coming from the right. She'd cut miles off the course. Padraig considered reporting her, but decided he could do without the hassle. (He told me her name and I'm tempted to write it down, but similarly don't need the bother. Plus I only have his word for it; if he made a mistake and I report it here, it's libel.) Anyway, we both agree, Padraig and I, that cheating in an ultra – cheating generally, but especially when you're not even in contention to win – is the most pointless exercise imaginable. We only run these races, most of us honest folk, for personal growth and satisfaction. Where does cheating come into that? If you've only run, say, 92 miles of a 100-mile race, how do you then look your fellow competitors and indeed yourself in the eye? Teachers tell you that if you cheat in an exam, you're only cheating yourself. But that's not strictly true is it? You're actually cheating everyone else. In an ultra, you really are only cheating yourself.

I admit to having witnessed something similar during a 50-mile race in some woods just north of London. Five 10-mile laps, and a bloke in front of me cut a good three miles and two significant climbs off one of them. What a complete loser, I thought at the time. And still do. I never saw his number or I'd have definitely said something.

Padraig tells me cheating is becoming an increasingly large problem in the USA. The sport is reeling from a fraudulent run across America. A Londoner called Rob Young is widely believed to have cut corners during an attempt to break the long-standing transcontinental record. The 3,000-mile run from Pacific to East Coast has stood at 46 days since 1980 despite numerous attempts to break it.

For several weeks Young was on course to smash the record. He was making it look easy … too easy. His daily mileage was, as one blogger put it at the time, 'unbelievable – and I mean that in the literal sense'. Suspicions grew. One runner claimed that he went to meet Young in rural Kansas only to find his RV driving slowly down the road with no runner in sight.

A group of experienced ultra-runners dubbing themselves 'The Geezers' decided to follow and observe, at which point the mileage plummeted from 70 or 80 miles a day to barely 40. They watched for five days and grew to respect Young's astonishing tenacity before he was eventually forced to call a halt to the challenge on medical grounds. He denies all allegations of cheating.

A full investigation was commissioned by his sponsors, and here is the sorry conclusion:

> The bottom line: The evidence that we reviewed for this investigation indicates that Rob Young received unauthorised assistance in his attempt to run across the United States. We have identified no alternative plausible explanation for the data-of-record other than assistance, most likely in the form of riding in or on a vehicle for large parts of the attempt.

Ever since, levels of paranoia in the US ultra scene have reached fever pitch. I'm depressed to learn from Padraig that other instances of cheating are on the rise. We do tend to follow America's lead in the UK don't we? Please not this. Like I said at the start, running these things is – or certainly should be – about feeding the good wolf. We definitely don't need big bad wolves huffing and puffing about the place.

If ever the good wolf was in evidence, the wolf representing joy, humility, compassion and hope, it was at Her Majesty's Prison Berwyn one October afternoon. Ever since I'd met (actually run into, literally, we almost knocked each other out) a young man called Ryan on Hammersmith Bridge, I'd had the idea that a prison run – for inmates in a prison – could be a Good thing. With a capital G.

Once we'd both recovered from the initial clash of heads, Ryan (not his real name) told me how running had basically kept him out of prison. How he'd always been in trouble at school, for fighting mostly, and how after one particular fight they said that's it, enough, and chucked him out.

Looking back, the way I was heading, I was maybe heading inside. I was angry all the time, looking for reasons to kick off and I didn't care about myself or anything. Negative. Horrible. Then my mate's uncle, he said I should try running. I didn't want to, and I didn't have any proper gear, but I'm glad I said yes. When I got back I realised I was pleased with myself, and maybe that was the first time, properly.

If running could help someone apparently on course for prison, I reasoned, surely it would also help those already serving time. Even if just to boost self-respect, and perhaps break a vicious circle of a lack of self-esteem. Then I met Erwin James, a convicted murderer and *Guardian* journalist. He was released in 2004 after serving 20 years of a life sentence. Whilst inside, he wrote a regular newspaper column and has since published several books. In fact I met him at an authors' event in central London, and although everyone around us was sipping wine and having intelligent literary conversations, Erwin and I had the germ of an idea of running round and round a prison yard.

It took quite some sorting, I can tell you. A lot of emails. But eventually, over two years later, we found ourselves in the main yard of the largest fully operational prison in the UK. Over 2,000 Category C male prisoners call Berwyn home. Two keen members of the Physical Education department had sorted the labyrinthine logistics and got the whole place enthused. Loads of people had signed up for the run and they'd decided to do it for charity, for BBC Children in Need. Pudsey came to prison for the day. There was a choice between a fancy dress, assault course-style 5K, with men and staff working in pairs, or a more serious 10K. I ran the longer race. It was an inspirational day. The Governor, Alun Johnson, a big Liverpool fan, is equally evangelical when he talks about the prison's values and how he subtly helps the men (not the prisoners, the men) focus on the future, not the past. Accommodation cells are called rooms, for instance, everything aiming to feel as normal as possible. How can you confidently look forwards if you keep being reminded of your past mistakes?

The runs are all part of this. Because when you're in prison – actually, wherever you are, but in prison it's more sharply focused – you need little wins. And going for a run is always, *always*, a win. Completing your first 10K, five laps around the outside perimeter of HMP Berwyn, surrounded by high fences topped with barbed wire, that's a significant win.

I ran much of the race with Steven, who had two years left to serve of a 16-year sentence. He has a lightning quick 5K PB, but had never run any further. After two laps he started to tire. But like my brother-in-law David, he can't abide being overtaken. I only wanted to move ahead because I thought having me panting and yapping away next to his left ear might be beginning to grate. However, every time I increased the pace and moved alongside, he sped up to keep me on his shoulder. This is a game I secretly enjoy playing with David (but only on the rare occasions I'm in better shape than he is; he's a head teacher, so usually at the end of a long term). Every few minutes I'll up the pace, forcing him to do the same if he wants to stay in front – which he always does. Trouble is, it tends to take longer to break him than I'd bargained for and I end up gasping for air and feeling a bit of a plonker.

Steven eventually let me pass and I began to soak in my surroundings. I was enthused to hear so much mutual encouragement. This culminated in Steven, who was first prisoner across the line, heading out for an extra loop to support a friend of his, the final finisher, throughout the last 2km. Everybody was applauded in, most loudly the guy who'd taken longest. Truly inspirational. The prison now has a Thursday Running Club hosted by the Governor and parkrun are simultaneously beginning to do their wonderful thing in prisons.

Padraig listens patiently as I recount my prison run experience in detail, then for some reason decides he has some faster running in his legs and powers ahead. It's the last I see of him. Over the next several miles, I alternately run with an Italian and a Mexican. Both auto-qualified* for the Spartathlon and are aiming for sub-30 hour

---

* You automatically get into the Spartathlon if you're 20% better than any of the dozen or so qualifying criteria. For instance, you need to have completed a 100-mile race in 21 hours to be eligible for the draw. If you've run a 100-miler in under 16:48, you can go straight into the following year's race with no need to bother with the lottery of the draw. Each country has only a certain number of places (it's 25 for the UK, 60 for Greece) so an auto-qualifier simply reduces the number of places each country has available in the draw. Most nations have waiting lists. It's a fiercely complicated process, the Spartathlon draw, and they make a televised event of it in early March. You don't receive an email (or anything) to let you know you've got in; you simply

finishing times. The fact that I'm with them as we approach halfway confirms my lingering suspicions that I've started too fast. I stop for some sustenance at an aid station as the Italian runs straight through. Meanwhile my Mexican friend, who's been slurring his words, suddenly slumps down into a chair. He's exhausted, spent. There's nothing I can do but leave him with the last of my caffeinated gels and my best wishes, and press on.

Through another checkpoint and I'm surprised and horrified to see Mick, my Aussie roommate, standing around despondently. Something must be going badly wrong; Mick should be a long way ahead.

It's his stomach. He can't run a step without needing the loo. Hence the constant farting of the past few days. By the time I catch up with him he's had to squat behind a bush a dozen times. Mick looks utterly disconsolate, as well he might. Brisbane to Athens is a long way to travel, only for your race to be ruined by some lingering food poisoning. I'd had a lengthy chat with a Greek pharmacist on his behalf the previous afternoon, and try to think back in case she'd said anything useful. But he's been following her advice, been taking the pills, and he's still suffering. We walk together for a while before Mick insists I run on. I do so with a heavy heart. Horrible way for a race to unravel, though not uncommon.

Meanwhile, almost guiltily, I'm still running strong. Fully 70 miles into the race and I'm feeling like Popeye after a can of spinach.

I've been reliably informed that very few people pull out after the mountain, so that's what I'm fixating on. *Just get to the top of the mountain*, I keep thinking, *and everything will be fine*. The summit is

---

check the website when you remember. In fact the only piece of communication you receive from the Spartathlon between submitting your entry in January and turning up on the start line in September is a terse email in mid May: *Dear Vassos, We inform you that your race (bib) number is: 7. Regards, the Spartathlon admin*. Everything else you glean from the website. It's all rather lovable. And the international flavour that the draw engenders only adds to the allure. The night before the race, I had dinner with a Malaysian, a Lithuanian, a Guatemalan and an Aussie.

around two-thirds of the way to Sparta, just over 100 miles into the race. The checkpoint cut-off times gradually ease thereafter. Away from the nagging worry about going too fast, at least I'm building a nice time buffer.

Ancient Nemea is where Hercules killed the Nemean Lion. Today you can still see the ruins of the temple to his father, the god Zeus. I'm lucky enough to arrive in the last of the daylight to properly appreciate its majesty. There's a party going on in the village centre, crews wait expectantly for their runners, locals mill about in the tavernas, but I struggle to enjoy the carnival atmosphere. As I run into the checkpoint, I suddenly realise I've lost my jacket. It's a wonderful thing, my waterproof jacket – lighter than air and it can fold into an astonishingly small bundle. Cost a fortune too, so I'm gutted to have lost it. The thought of turning back for it briefly enters my mind, though it could be many thousands of footsteps which need retracing.

The crews helping out the British runners are conspicuous for the same bright red T-shirts with a quotation from the Spartathlon's founder, John Foden: 'I shan't wish you luck because if you have trained properly, you won't need luck. And if you haven't trained properly, then luck will be of no use.'

Well, I'm in luck. A friend of a friend is crewing for one of the Brits, and asks if there's anything I need (they were all amazingly kind to me, the British crews. As were the Greek volunteers at each and every aid station). When I tell Russ about the lost waterproof shell, he races to his hire car and produces one of his own running shirts for me to borrow – *in case it gets chilly*, he says. Which it soon will.

I leave Nemea in higher spirits than when I arrived. As evening falls I'm hiking up a deserted farm track. For the moment there are no other runners around me. I revel in the darkness and solitude. I break into a trot up the gentle gradient and a faintly risible fantasy takes hold: I am Pheidippides, racing to Sparta to save civilisation! Dusk turns to night and still I continue running upwards, just like the famous messenger 2,500 years before me, perhaps even up this very hill. It starts to rain,

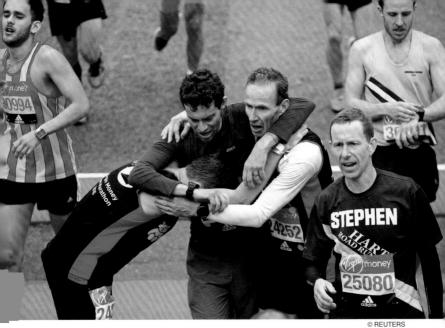

▲ Compare and contrast... Breaking three hours in the
London Marathon – we look like castaways!

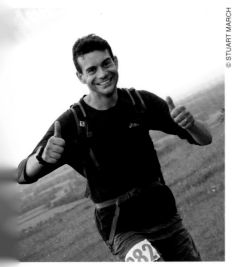

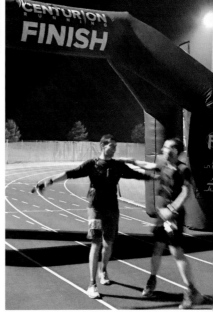

... A few weeks later, all smiles as
I run my first 100-mile race across
the beautiful South Downs.

There's no nice way of putting this, endurance running does disgusting things to your toes!

▼ Iconic starts to epic races. Serenaded by a Welsh Male Voice Choir in Conwy Castle as we head into the wild, trackless mountains.

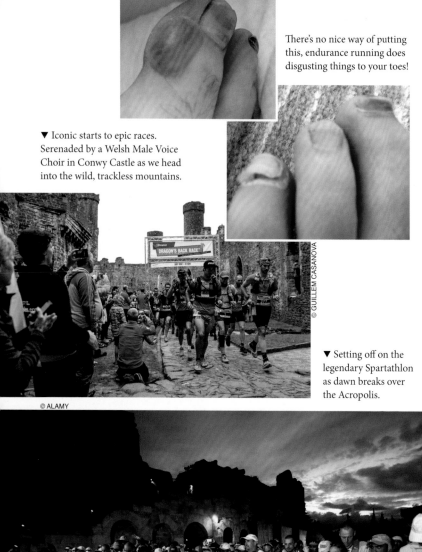

© GUILLEM CASANOVA

© ALAMY

▼ Setting off on the legendary Spartathlon as dawn breaks over the Acropolis.

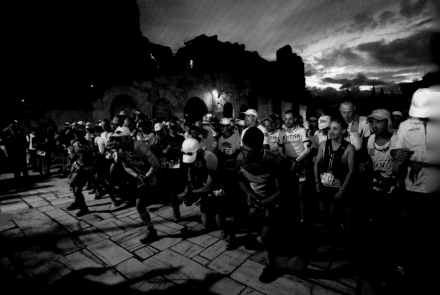

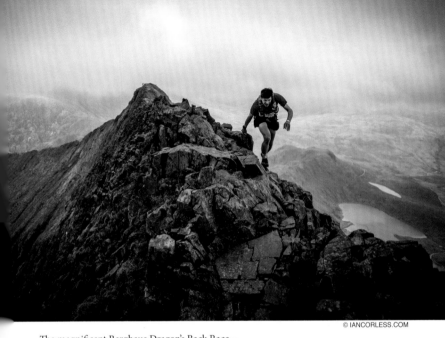

The magnificent Berghaus Dragon's Back Race –
five days along the mountainous spine of Wales.
Spectacular scenery. Treacherous footing. Really hard.

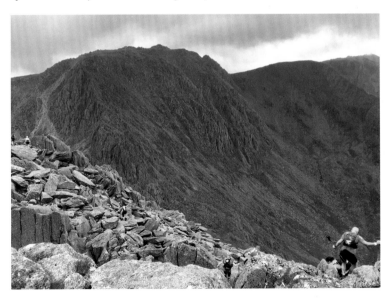

It's been my immense privilege to talk to some of the world's greatest endurance runners. In every case, astonishing running prowess is matched by kindness and humility.

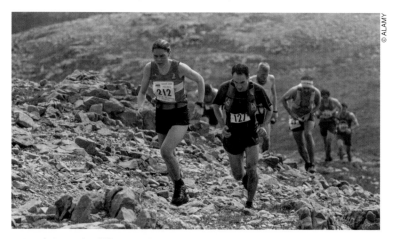

© ALAMY

▲ Jasmin Paris, elite fell runner, Skyrunning champion and multiple record holder.

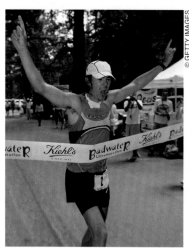

© GETTY IMAGES

▲ The great Scott Jurek, one of the world's most dominant endurance runners and famously committed to a plant-based diet.

▶ Mimi Anderson, an inspiration to so many, generous and enthusiastic even as she comes to terms with injury.

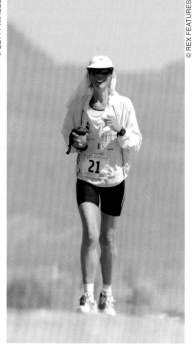

© REX FEATURES

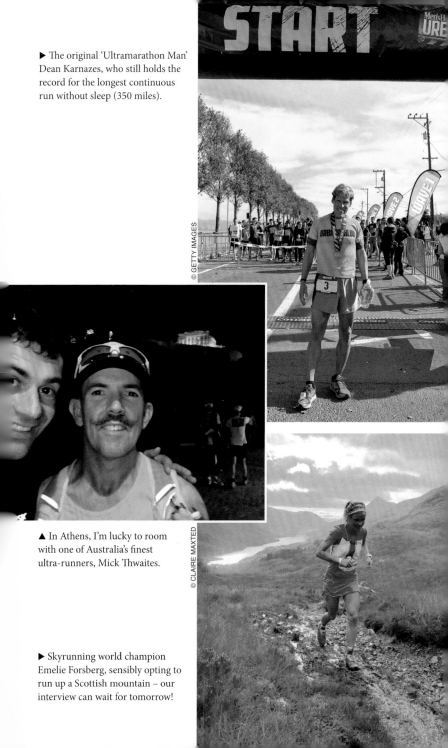

▶ The original 'Ultramarathon Man' Dean Karnazes, who still holds the record for the longest continuous run without sleep (350 miles).

© GETTY IMAGES

© CLAIRE MAXTED

▲ In Athens, I'm lucky to room with one of Australia's finest ultra-runners, Mick Thwaites.

▶ Skyrunning world champion Emelie Forsberg, sensibly opting to run up a Scottish mountain – our interview can wait for tomorrow!

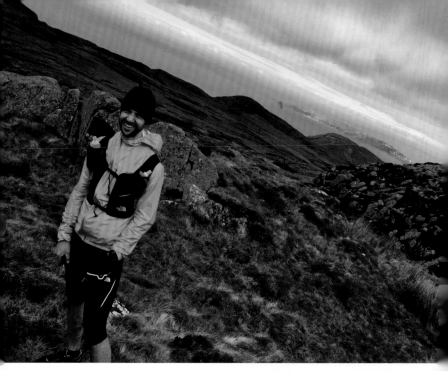

▲ Happy training days... In Snowdonia with UTMB winner Jez Bragg – on his birthday!

▶ With brother-in-law Dave, giving our dogs a headteacherly pep talk ahead of a long run in the Downs.

▼ Marcus Scotney wins the Dragon's Back Race but his beagle Sherlock, on Cadar Idris summit, grabs all the adulation (and Instagram followers!)

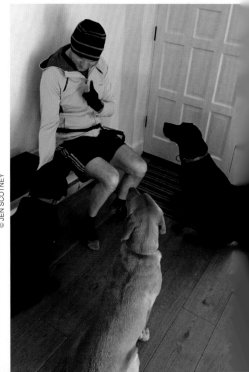

© JEN SCOTNEY

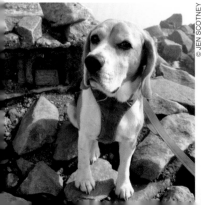

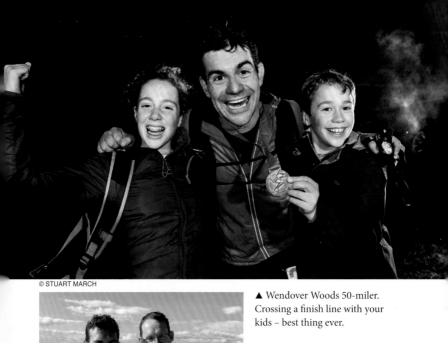

▲ Wendover Woods 50-miler. Crossing a finish line with your kids – best thing ever.

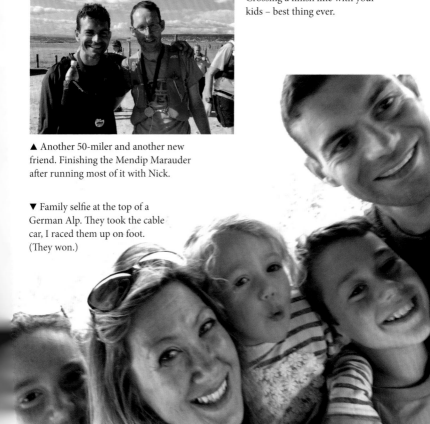

▲ Another 50-miler and another new friend. Finishing the Mendip Marauder after running most of it with Nick.

▼ Family selfie at the top of a German Alp. They took the cable car, I raced them up on foot. (They won.)

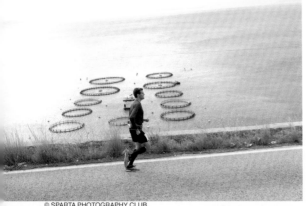

◄ The long, long, long road to Sparta. 153 historic miles of city, mountain, olive groves and seaside.

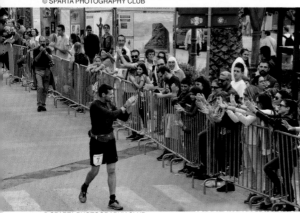

◄ But the atmosphere when you get there is immense. Truly humbling.

▼ I kissed a foot. (And I liked it.)

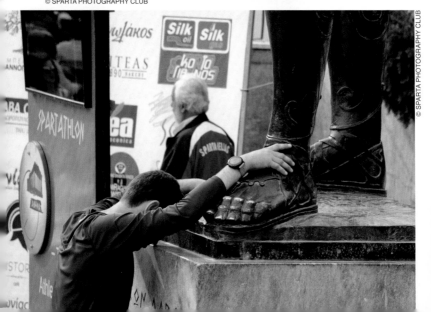

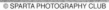

ever so gently, almost imperceptibly; I can smell the moisture rather than feel it. It's pitch dark now, there's no light coming from the moon, and even though I can scarcely see my hand in front of my face, all my other senses seem supercharged. I am Pheidippides, I have a critical purpose – and I am invincible!

I trip over a rock and land unceremoniously on my arse, bloodying my shoulder in the process. Digging out my head torch dissipates any lingering notion that I'm a messenger on a mission. *Just reach the top of the mountain*, I repeat to myself. *And stop being an idiot.*

The night-time hours of the Spartathlon are perhaps the most magical of all. We run through remote villages where residents are having parties in our honour. Tavernas throw open their doors. Kids run alongside us wanting autographs. From the oldest *yiayia* (grandmother) sitting on her balcony dressed in the traditional black, to couples and young families eating and drinking in the village squares, everyone shouts encouragement and applauds as we go past. If we doubted it before, here's the proof: this race really is a big deal in Greece.

More proof. We're mostly following painted arrows on the streets to guide us, but there are many permanent road signs also pointing the way, brown with yellow lettering: *Spartathlon, In the Footsteps of Pheidippides, 246km, Athens to Sparta*. There must be 50 of them between the two cities. These signs are redundant on 364 days of the year, but the race is so important, they've put them up just for this one day every 12 months. Christmas lights get more use every December than these signs have ever had.

Lyrkia is a picturesque little village at the bottom of the mountain. Again there are ancient ruins to be admired but it's late evening when I arrive and I don't see them. It's raining harder now and despite the extra T-shirt, I'm starting to get really cold. I ask for a bin bag at the aid station and fashion it into a makeshift waterproof coat. My legs still feel strong. It's a steady climb now to the mountain base, then 3,500 feet to the summit. *Just get to the top of the mountain*, I tell myself for the hundredth time.

Dean Karnazes is the self-styled, original Ultramarathon Man. He ran these very hills a year or two before me and wrote a book, *The Road to Sparta*, about his quest to conquer the Spartathlon. His first book, *Confessions of an All-Night Runner*, inspired many to take up the sport. He holds the world record for running the furthest without sleep, 350 miles in 80 hours. He's run a marathon in each of the 50 states on 50 consecutive days. He's won Badwater, the Vermont Trail 100-mile race, and once ran 148 miles in 24 hours on a treadmill. He's also, just at this very moment, a bit cross with me. I'm 10 minutes late having been stuck in traffic. I'm effusively apologetic, which seems to do the trick.

This is a few months before the Spartathlon and the race has been dominating my thoughts and training. I ask him how it feels to finish – what goes through your head when, after 153 miles of unrelenting effort, you arrive at the giant statue of the warrior king Leonidas in Sparta and complete your quest by touching – or traditionally, charmingly, by kissing – his foot.

Dean pauses for a second, says he needs to get his head in that place. I suggest it might be something akin to joy, ecstasy? I tell him how it felt when I finished my first 100-mile race, how the bubble of contentment stayed with me for weeks and reminded me of the emotions I experienced when my children were born.

Absolutely. At the flash point of the finish line, at that moment, there's always a burst of adrenaline and I've seen it in others as well. No matter how tough it's been, when you see that finish line, there's always some elation and there's excitement, adrenaline. Then in the moment following that, there's typically a lot of fatigue, a lot of pain, and there are physical feelings of both euphoria as well as misery.

Then it gradually becomes exactly what you explained and the experience itself somehow, it elevates larger than the trivialities of everyday life, like having a kid. I think that's a good analogy, where there's something that lingers that says, wow, this was a really special experience that is beyond my day to day getting stuck in traffic, like you just did – and being late for appointments. So, I couldn't agree more with what you said.

I take the renewed dig at my tardiness in the spirit in which it was intended. Playfully, I hope, but also perhaps a little reminder. Here is a man not to be messed with. After all, he's broken some of the most impressive endurance records of all time. He's introduced many thousands to long distance running. I find myself wondering what Dean does to get through the tough times on a long run? What mental tricks does he play?

I try not to play mental tricks. I try instead to be in the moment of time. I've tried chanting mantras and I've tried trying to put my head some place else, but those don't work. Inevitably, you say, 'I'm just doing this because I'm in such pain, I'm trying to trick myself to get through it.' Instead, I just focus on being in the here and now, being in the present moment of time. So not thinking about how much further there is to go or not reflecting on the past, just thinking about putting your next footstep in front of your last to the best of your abilities. So really getting very granular and just saying, 'I will take my next step to the best of my ability and then the next step.' Just focus on the very moment of time and don't think of anything else. If you can do that, if you can get your head there, you're almost going to a Zen-like place where you're just moving in space and time. You're not thinking about the misery you're in. You're not thinking about the many miles and miseries ahead. You're just thinking about being the best you can right then and there.

This is something you hear again and again from ultra-runners. From all runners, come to think of it. Running as mindfulness. I remember back to that day in Keswick after the extraordinary boat trip to the start line. It was my first time running in the fells (mountains) of the Lake District. I crested that first peak on a sublime spring morning, and all of England seemed spread out before me. My senses were in overdrive.

My breathing was loud, long and lustrous. All pain and exhaustion were washed clean away as I realised there was nowhere else I'd rather be in that moment, nothing else I'd prefer to be doing. Is this mindfulness what Dean loves most about ultra-running?

Absolutely. To me, that's very cleansing. It's rejuvenating because throughout the course of the day, our lives are frenetic. There's a lot of shit happening. Just like you've just experienced. As well, you're probably getting emails coming in and people are calling you. You're trying to monitor your Twitter feed, but when you're doing these races of great duration, there's none of that.

All that stuff becomes just noise in the background and you have this clarity of purpose. It's just get to the finish line. I have one goal for maybe 24, maybe 48 hours, just one thing, and that is just to keep moving forward. I think that I'm very drawn to it. I'm very introverted and to me, that experience of just being by myself and having that solidarity of focus, like I said, it's rejuvenating.

Born to Run is kind of the sacred script of ultra-running. It's good. I'm sure Dean has read it (and he has). He initially planned to run to Sparta wearing the traditional footwear and attire of the Ancient Greek messenger though I don't think he managed it in the end; I think he wore a modern running vest and shoes. I'm keen to get his opinion on the thorny issue of barefoot running. In the book, Christopher McDougall, a former war correspondent, explores the little-known world of the Mexican Tarahumara, a tribe of extraordinary athletes who still live as they have done for hundreds of years in the Copper Canyons of Central America. And boy, can they run. Extreme distances, in extreme heat, over extreme terrain – not a problem for these supreme athletes, who glide over the ground, fuelled mainly by chia seeds, as though they were being poured over the terrain.

McDougall suggests (slash proves, depending on your point of view) that we humans were indeed, as the title of his book suggests, born to run. That we used to chase down prey across the African savannah until the antelope, say, collapsed through exhaustion. We have the extra endurance, because we thermo-regulate; we sweat like no other species. Persistence hunting, it's called, and there's evidence to suggest it was the most efficient way for primitive man to kill prey. That's why we look like we do, and not like Neanderthal Man, who was stronger, faster, more savage – but less canny, less able to simply keep on running. There's definitely something in this. When I run, especially on trail rather than tarmac, I feel somehow that I'm doing right by my genes.

Furthermore, McDougall suggests (slash proves) that modern running shoes are the cause of many of today's running injuries. That we were meant to run barefoot, or as close to that as possible – the Tarahumara use just basic sandals, flip-flops really, thin strips of leather under the soles of their feet with a thin cord tied around the toes and ankle. Sticking a great gel cushion on the heel of our shoes, the argument goes, is merely altering our natural gait, prompting a heel (rather than mid-foot) ground strike – and that's where niggles and injuries are often traced to. Our lavishly cushioned shoes are effectively doing the opposite of what the manufacturers are promising.

A Harvard evolutionary biologist called Daniel Lieberman looked into this. He went to the Copper Canyon to compare traditional sandal-wearing runners with some of the younger Tarahumara men and women who've grown up in Western-style shoes. Many of the famously shy Tarahumara refused to be filmed, but a dozen agreed to be part of the study. The findings 'suggest that the Tarahumara who wear huaraches (sandals) have stronger intrinsic muscles that lead to a stiffer longitudinal arch'. This could of course lead to fewer injuries, in theory, but Lieberman was keen not to draw too many conclusions. You get the feeling he gets fed up with us runners taking bits of his research and, well, running with it.

> Finally, it is worth considering the relevance of these results for
> the majority of runners who grow up wearing shoes, rarely if
> ever run ultra-marathons, and are habituated to conventional

89

running shoes. Evidence that traditional Tarahumara who wear huaraches mostly avoid rear-foot landings on flat surfaces at moderate speeds is hardly justification for someone to switch to minimal shoes and stop heel striking.

Personally, I agree that barefoot running is more natural. Probably better all-round. But that said, I still wear the same trusty shoe with a great big mattress underneath it – and I'm loathe to change. If it ain't broke and all that. I also believe the gait is more important than the shoe. But I wonder whether Dean buys into McDougall's *Born to Run* theory.

Yeah, I do, very much so. I know Chris and in my most recent book about the Spartathlon, I talk about the Ancient Greek foot messengers, even pre-dating the Tarahumara. And these guys were running hundreds of miles across Southern Greece, a very rocky mountainous terrain, very effectively.

So there's that example and they were pretty well trained. They were very sophisticated for athletes 2,500 years ago. Then there's the argument that we've evolved into the apex predator, if you will, because of our ability to locomote long distances and to chase down prey over great distances.

Final question, Dean: If you had one story that encapsulates your life as the Ultramarathon Man, what would it be and why?

This is probably not going to be what you're expecting, but I've run on all seven continents of earth twice over. I've run in some of the most remote and exotic places imaginable, the Gobi Desert, Atacama, Namibia. But the run that sticks with me the most is a 10K. And the reason is I ran the 10K with my daughter, Alexandria, on her tenth birthday. I don't know why that supersedes everything else I've done, but there's something about her and I clicking on that run, and me seeing her in a different light.

So Alexandria was 10 and we're running this 10K together and at probably kilometre 8, she was really hurting. She was in that place where I can just tell she was in a ton of pain. She's a 10-year-old and I'm thinking, 'Okay, she's going to stop at any step.' I was just about to turn to her and say, 'You know, Alexandria, I'm so proud of you for making it this far. We can try again. We can try another 10K at some point.' Right when I was going to tell her that because I thought she was going to stop, she turned to me and said, 'Dad, I can do this,' and just sprinted. I couldn't even keep up with her the last kilometre.

To see your child through different eyes and realise, 'Wow, this is a person that is somewhat like me on a different sort of level.' I don't know. That seems to transcend everything else I've done.

Which is a lovely way to end our chat. Or it would've been if Dean hadn't decided to be even nicer and add how much he likes us Brits.

It's funny. I have a big following in the UK and I love it there. It's not a place I necessarily would pick as my top destination, but I've just grown to love it. There's a fondness I have for the people, I think, more than anything else.

Perhaps that means I've been forgiven for being late.

Back in Greece, I'm blissfully early. I arrive at the checkpoint before the mountain base and work out that I've built a buffer of almost five hours. I allow myself a moment of optimism. I still feel fine, I'm about to climb the mountain, I'm hours ahead of where I need to be, and as everyone keeps telling me, hardly anyone drops out after the mountain. For the first time all race, indeed for the first time since I entered the ballot to get in, I believe I'll probably make it to Sparta. What can possibly go wrong?

Little do I know.

9. merthyr

I'm commentating at the darts. Just love the darts. I'm also running in the Brecon Beacons. This has every chance of turning into basically the perfect day!

It's before dawn on the morning of the second-ever Champions League of Darts in Cardiff. I'm there for BBC TV, but I've got nothing to do until the first match on the oche at 1:30pm. Two weeks out from the Spartathlon, I decide a long run is in order and check the map on my phone for the nearest bit of green. As I swipe and wipe, a very large bit of green emerges directly north of the Welsh capital: the Brecon Beacons.

I've never run in the Brecons before, having failed to make it that far south during the Dragon's Back Race. It's still dark outside so I check the clock to see if I can reasonably get up yet. Ten minutes to six – perfect. It'll just be getting light by the time I've driven to centre of the National Park. As an extra treat, a special surprise given that this is Wales – it's miraculously not raining.

Thirty glorious miles later, I pass the town of Merthyr Tydfil and suddenly the Brecons surround me in all their splendour. A watery, pink sun is starting to burn off the dawn mist forming in the valleys. In the car I need fog lights, but now and again the mist clears to offer a glimpse of the spectacular scenery up above. I'd been meaning to drive to the foot of Pen y Fan, find a public car park and set off on some well-trodden routes up the highest peak in South Wales. On a whim, because I can't contain my excitement a moment longer, I take the first turning I see up a small track, dump the car and just start running. Not so much onwards and upwards, as upwards and upwards. I'm desperate to see what's up there, keen to immerse myself in what is apparently one of the most bewitching landscapes in Britain. Pen y Fan can wait.

I approach a gate with a charming handwritten sign hung around it: 'Private land. Take nothing but photos. Leave nothing but footprints. And please don't let your dog chase our sheep!'

Up the path, legs pumping, arms swinging, climbing, climbing... my dog would love it here, I think. But she's back at home whilst I'm puffing up this unforgiving slope. It's always difficult to start an early run with a prolonged uphill, but the benefits are massive. All future terrain feels light and easy, even the climbs. It's like the legs go bionic. Which is exactly what happens as I hop over a stile, the path levels out and I'm in the Beacons.

I survey the glorious scene before me and whoop with happiness. Literally whoop. A sheep surveys me oddly. But then she's used to these views; I do most of my running in London. Not many sparkling reservoirs nestling in lush valleys on the Edgware Road. Hyde Park is lovely enough, but you'll do well to spot any hilltop cairns among the bridleways. And clifftop castle ruins are few and far between on Hammersmith Bridge.

I'm running along a grassy path, which promptly disappears into heather and bog. I come to a stop. I'm wearing road running shoes, new ones, and I'm not keen to get them and my feet soaking wet. Options are: back the way I've just come, or soggy socks. Tricky. I'm not a fan of turning back during a run (is anyone?) but I really don't want wet feet and *really* don't want to spoil the shoes I've just bought ahead of a 153-mile run on dodgy Greek pavements. I'll need all the cushioning I can get. Plus, I don't want to get lost. This is remote and untamed countryside, I remind myself, and I don't have any useful equipment beyond a mobile phone. Currently there's a good signal (I do check), but I certainly ought to be careful.

I turn back, and after a few hundred yards veer off the path along a small sheep trod winding its way towards some rocks. But before long, the trod itself becomes sodden. I pause again, then turn back once more.

I lose my bearings as I skip over shin-deep grass and heather, trying to avoid slipping up or twisting an ankle in one of the mysterious, deep hollows in the terrain. Anything vaguely resembling a grassy path or even a trod becomes a memory. I dither. This is a wild and trackless Welsh mountain. What did I expect, having only recently competed in the wildest and trackless-est mountain race in the world, encompassing these very hills, only three months ago? Truth is, I've gone soft again. Funny how fast that can happen when the most savage terrain you experience is Wimbledon Common. Or when you turn off the Tamsin Trail, the main cycle and walking path around Richmond Park, and feel adventurous. I urgently need to get a grip.

Sometimes in life, exactly the right thing happens at exactly the right moment. As I stand there feeling very city-soft on those radiant yet menacing hills, my phone pings. A text from Kílian Jornet, the world's finest mountain runner, asking if now is a good time to chat. (Just to be clear, despite my job, this sort of thing doesn't happen very often. It's a huge thrill to get a text from Kílian.) He's in town – or rather, the highlands of Scotland – for the Salomon Glen Coe Skyline race, and when we'd been due to speak yesterday, he was up a mountain with his girlfriend. She is the equally amazing ultra-runner Emelie Forsberg, and I'd been due to interview them both. Not that they'd known anything about it. Before they could be told, Emelie was off trying her luck in the notorious 'vertical kilometre', and Kílian went along to support. A thousand metres of height gain in less than 5km, a leg-burning, lung-busting ascent from sea level to Munro summit. It takes some competitors almost three hours to complete; Forsberg breezed up in a little over 50 minutes – and that was merely by way of a warm-up for the main event, the Skyline itself – a truly brutal 55km race with 5,000 metres of climbing.

Back in Wales, I wonder when Emelie Forsberg or Kílian Jornet last worried about getting their feet wet whilst running. I think about asking them, but bottle it. I call Emelie's mobile. I love the fact that we'll be speaking while she's in the Scottish Highlands, and I'm in the Brecon Beacons – and that the focus of the whole weekend for me, the wallpaper, is darts. About as far away from mountain running as it's possible for sport to be. I consider asking her about darts too, but again think better of it. Probably for the best – she seems charming and happy, but focused. Instead I ask how she's enjoying Scotland.

I'm really happy to be here in Glen Coe because the mountains are like the perfect mix between Norwegian and Swedish mountains, so I feel really at home. But it's also completely new for me. I have such a good feeling to be here and explore these beautiful mountains and their culture and the villages – it's super-cool.

The previous evening, a mutual friend emailed me a picture of Emelie running the vertical kilometre. Despite the gradient, she looked ridiculously serene and utterly content, grinning away under the trademark flower in her hair.

Yeah, I was happy. In my element. I just… love running. And I love mountains. I started to realise that I really was a passionate mountain runner a decade or so ago, when I turned 20. But I didn't start to compete for another five years because I just didn't need it and I wasn't introduced to racing. So I'm still pretty new to competing even though I've been getting a kick out of running in the mountains for many years now. Also, I'm just so grateful that I can run, that I am able to do what I'm doing. Even though it might be hurting, that's bigger than the suffering.

Emelie has a famously infectious jubilance about her. She burst onto the mountain running scene at the 2011 European Skyrunning Championships in the Italian Dolomites, where she won two gold medals and a silver. A few months previously, she'd been almost completely unknown.

At that time, the ultra-running press (such as it is) was ablaze with articles about this bright new star with her simple love of nature. 'Forsberg's running successes are not the primary goal it seems, rather a simple by-product of her deep-rooted love for moving fast in the mountains, and, damn, does she move fast,' eulogised runner/writer Robbie Lawless after she told him about her beliefs and priorities.

Racing has only recently been part of my life. Nature and my passion for being outside have always been there and I would not let anything take away that passion. Running, skiing, climbing, walking, gardening, farming – that's who I am. That is how I define myself. I don't define myself as a racer or competitor. But yes, I love winning of course, it's big, but at the same time it doesn't matter at all.

That's something I'm keen to explore whilst I've got her on the phone. I'm lucky enough to meet a large number of elite sportspeople and very few have this level of maturity, awareness or perspective. I tell her how I'd been struggling with the boggy ground in Wales. Does she ever struggle to find enjoyment in her running?

All runs are perfect in a way. You just need to see the perfection I think, and I'm pretty good at seeing what's really good, and appreciating it. So, it can't be everything – and can't be nothing. Like I mentioned before, it's really appreciating that I can do this. I don't ever take it for granted. If I'm tired during a race, I just think that tiredness, it's a small part. I should simply be happy with what I'm doing and grateful. That's what I think about if I start to feel tired or unmotivated. It's like I can just appreciate that I actually can be there.

You just need to live in the moment, right here and right now. And then you create a relationship with nature that makes you want to take care of it. One way for me to be able to do that, to take care of nature, is to eat seasonally and eat from my garden and don't eat meat and be a bit more conscious about what I'm doing and why I'm doing it.

Back in Wales, I'm already beginning to appreciate my surroundings more, whatever the state of my shoes and socks. And feeling a little guilty not to think things through like Emelie does – well basically, ever. I can't remember the last time I made my food choices based on seasonality. I inwardly decide to start. In the meantime, since she's brought up the subject of food... 'Emelie, what do you eat for breakfast?'

Forsberg is big into her food. She used to work in a bakery but now grows much of what she eats. She's long wanted to be self-sufficient and farms all manner of veggies and herbs in the garden of the house she shares with Jornet in Norway. Her smallholding even has its own Instagram account. 'With a shovel in my hands and dirt under my nails – that's when I feel really alive and connected to the earth.'

She says she's frequently been told she 'doesn't look like a runner' and once famously wrote a blog on body image which concluded with the words, 'Love your hips, breasts, butt and belly. The fat keeps you warm. And healthy.' She claims she has a very sweet tooth and that everything's OK in moderation. Everything natural, that is.

I have a pretty big garden and a small farm and, same as mountain running, it's a way in which I can be connected to nature. I take time to prepare my garden and to eat my food, and everything is connected. You just need to take the time to appreciate it.

And muesli is the breakfast of choice apparently. Or, if she's going on an early training run, just an organic bar – nuts and seeds – and a large cup of coffee. The bars will also feature tomorrow morning before she calmly obliterates both the field and the course record with that trademark flower in her hair. She'll win the Glen Coe Skyline and throughout almost eight hours' hard running, she'll seem to smile serenely. She helps organise the Tromsø SkyRace, part of the same series, and perhaps prefers the simpler, running-only perspective.

Yeah, I'm super-happy to be here. It's a truly amazing race in Scotland with a lot of technical parts, almost climbing, scrambling, so I'm really looking forward to doing it. I'm excited to see how I'm going to be feeling after a few hours of running because I haven't been able to train over long distances. It's going to be a super-exciting day.

So many things motivate me. I have two competing seasons: winter and summer. That motivates me to be a better skier, a better runner, and also to improve all my capabilities, to say that I can be as good as I can be in every kind of discipline and distance. That motivates me.

She passes the phone to the other half of the sport's star couple. Kílian Jornet is widely considered to be the finest ultra-distance and mountain runner on the planet. When we speak he's just become the fastest man in history to climb the north face of Everest. In fact he did it twice in a week, without the aid of oxygen or fixed ropes. Then he rushed straight back to Europe and claimed victory in a hotly contested Marathon du Mont Blanc. From Himalayas to Alps, and next to the San Juan mountains of Colorado for the iconic, 100-mile Hardcore Trail, one of the most famous races on the ultra calendar. Which he won for the fourth time in a row only to return to Europe for the Ultra-Trail de Mont-Blanc (UTMB).

The 2017 edition was widely regarded as the trail race with the deepest elite field. Anywhere. Ever. Jornet finished a close second to the Frenchman François D'Haene. After his exertions that summer he was on a hiding to nothing, but says he simply wanted to be there 'because there was a high standard and I wanted to enjoy real competition with the best runners in the world. François had a great race and he deserved to win.'

So what on earth's he doing only a few days later, about to compete again in Glen Coe against another stellar field?

Yeah, I just like to compete. The main thing is I like to run – and I like to run different things, like long or short, technical or flat – whatever. What I like about competing is to test yourself all the time, because it keeps you motivated for training. It keeps you motivated for training hard and pushing the limits and I think that's fun. I think it's like a kid's game, like you are with friends and you want to be the winner. Also you want to have fun and just put yourself in the mountains.

The Welsh wind whips though my thin running shirt and I shiver. I'm feeling increasingly sheepish about my lamentable early efforts in the Beacons. I wonder where the word 'sheepish' comes from, because the sheep all around me look more bored than embarrassed. They've long since lost interest in the man in the black shorts and orange shirt who was recently running in weird stop-start circles but for the past 15 minutes has been standing around talking animatedly. On the other end of the phone of course, is someone who's basically the opposite of 'ooh, I want to keep my shoes all shiny and I don't want wet socks'. Kílian is mountain running; I'm darts. But it's rubbing off. There's a real joy about Jornet.

First, you have to love what you are doing, and to love being outside. And that's me. My passion is to be outside and to be running and to be climbing. So that's bigger than the pain. Occasionally something will come up and of course, in that moment it's painful and it can be hard. But looking at it another way, it's what I love to do and the motivation of discovering, it's much bigger.

What do you think about, Kílian, while you're running?

It can be many, many things. When you are running on an easy trail you can be training but thinking about what things you've got to do, like some work for example. It's the same as when you are sitting in front of the computer, you are thinking about daily things. Other times, if you are running on a very technical terrain, you need to do something creative in the movement, concentrating hard where you put your feet, where you put your hands, so it's kind of a meditation.

I don't like to look to the past. I always like to look to the future and in a way, it's easy to keep motivated when you're running in beautiful places because every morning is like, looking through the window, seeing nice mountains and saying, 'OK, I want to climb this summit and I want to explore this region.' Then you come to the summit and you see all the other mountains behind – and you think to yourself you want to go to the next one and the next one. So tomorrow I will go there. Because I love to be in the mountains. I love to run on the hill, and being on that hill is not like hard work or tough training for me. It's more like just fun. It's just nice to be outside.

My favourite run is the one I will run tomorrow. It's because that is what you are doing, it's the next thing. The important thing is to take the beauty of every place you are running. You can be running in the desert and it's beautiful and you embrace that, and you can be running here in Scotland and you embrace the landscape. Yeah, every place it has its own beauty and it's just exciting to see different things. Here, actually, the good thing is it's pretty open terrain. It's low vegetation, so you can run everywhere; you don't need to be on the trails to run because it's all just open mountains, so we have a freedom of choice that is incredible. And these combined with the ridges, and the scrambling... it's the perfect terrain for fell running.

He could just as easily be talking about where I'm standing 500 miles and an 8-hour drive due south. Well, the bit about no trails and open terrain anyway. There aren't so many scrambling ridges here. Strange as it may seem, given that I'm chatting to two of my heroes, I find myself keen to get off the phone and continue running. Just a couple more questions first.

I wonder which of his many achievements he's proudest of. I know I'm speaking to an extremely modest man but surely, just occasionally, he'll look back at something he's accomplished and think – *Wow, I'm quite pleased with that*. Whether it's a race victory or his best-selling book, *Run or Die*. Or perhaps the Summits of My Life project, in which he bids to set ascent and descent records for the most important mountains on the planet, culminating in the recent double-whammy up Everest. And surely he's proud of sticking to his renowned values, the seven rules for a purist and minimalist understanding of mountains, which underpin the Summits adventures.

I think I am proud of being polyvalent, versatile, more than achieving a single thing. But I've been able to do some good stuff in skiing and also in long-distance running, in mountaineering and vertical kilometres... So a good season for me is when I have done OK in races over different distances and terrains, more than having one big win in one particular big race.

Final thing then, Kílian. One more run before you die: where would it be?

If I had one more run…. Well you know, I'm a pretty practical person so probably if I had only one more run I would start running now, here in Glen Coe, but I would never stop. So I will just run and run and run around the world. I would just keep running.

An excellent answer. And it's exactly what I start doing in Wales. I thank Kílian and simply start running. Within seconds, I've stepped through a bog and disappeared up to my shins. I remember back to Snowdonia; it's just the sort of thing that happens to you in the Welsh mountains. A few months ago, I thought nothing of spending 16 hours running in soaking socks. I cross another stile and speed up as I run over some splashy, short grass towards what looks like a yellow flag in the distance.

I crest the hill, and start laughing. At myself. It *is* a yellow flag. It's billowing in the freshening breeze at the top of a thin white flagpole which in turn is stuck into a hole about 10cm wide. 10.8cm wide to be precise. I know this for a fact because the hole is in the middle of a patch of very short, well-maintained grass, and behind it is a large sandy crater.

Whilst I've been fretting about the wilderness and remoteness, checking whether I have a phone signal in case of emergency and steeling myself to run through soggy terrain – I've been on a golf course! Specifically Merthyr Tydfil Golf Course, which I later learn has 13 of its holes within the boundary of the Brecon Beacons National Park. But even so, a golf course. Where doubtless the first four balls of the weekend will soon be appearing, gloves on one hand and pushing clubs on trolleys. Apart from the obvious hazard of flying balls, a golf course is probably the least menacing landscape imaginable.

Sometimes, I conclude as I run on, trying to discern where the golf course ends and the Beacons begin, sometimes I genuinely do despair of myself.

10. winchester

A photo pings loudly onto the screen of my phone.

I'm five minutes into my first 100-mile race, and wonder who could be texting me just after 6am on a Saturday morning. This is the start of the iconic South Downs Way 100. We've just run around a field near Winchester and are about to be let loose onto the famous trail that a hundred hilly miles later will land us in Eastbourne.

I'd set the alarm at home in London for a quarter to three and crept about the house as quietly as possible, desperately trying not to wake the kids or – worse – the dog, who'd either bark in excitement and wake the kids anyway, or give me that doleful look which means 'you're wearing running shorts – please can I come along too?' Very difficult to refuse that look (she uses a similar trick to beg for food) but today she most certainly can't come along. Even Holly our mega Labrador might struggle to run a hundred miles in one go.

As, more to the point, might I. The furthest I've run before is 62, so this is quite a leap. The only thing I definitely know is to eat. And keep eating. For someone as greedy as me, it's paradise!

I'd learned my lesson in previous endurance events, notably a woefully undernourished Ironman triathlon. I was attempting the 112-mile bike section wearing cargo shorts (don't ask!), and on a whim after the 2.4-mile swim, decided to put all the food I'd prepared into one of the front pockets. Only trouble was, after treating myself to a nibble halfway around the bike course, I must have failed to put the food – actually a slightly odd-looking superfood cake of my own devising – back in the pocket properly. Because when I next looked for it in the transition tent before the run, it simply wasn't there.

Which was a bit of a blow, to be honest, as my stomach had long since begun rejecting the only other source of calories on offer, the gels being handed out at the aid stations. I was dizzy with hunger by the time I started running the marathon, and it's still probably the hardest thing I've ever completed. Even at the end of a triathlon, the marathon should have taken me no more than three and a half hours; it took five and a quarter. 315 minutes of unremitting, unbendable misery. Bonking, they call it, when you simply run out of petrol, your carbohydrate stores are depleted and you hit the wall. That day, the wall was 26.2 miles long.

So like I say, I definitely know enough to cram in as much food as I can – even in the kitchen in the middle of the night. It's 3am, I'm craving sleep but stuffing my face instead. Oats, toast with peanut butter, an apple, a protein ball, malt loaf loaded with butter, half a banana, a nutty breakfast bar…. Actually, who needs sleep? I find I could get used to this nocturnal gluttony… the other half of the banana, some Greek yoghurt and some porridge to finish.

I pack my running rucksack – mostly with more food to be honest, but also a head torch, waterproof jacket and other mandatory kit – and just when I'm congratulating myself on successfully leaving the house without waking anyone, I open the front door onto my toe. The inadvertent obscenity that escapes my mouth wakes most of the street. Under these circumstances I decide the best course of action, the honourable thing to do, the manly thing, is to run away as fast as possible before my wife gets downstairs. So I jump in the car and I've driven about a mile from home when I realise that I'm still wearing socks – and my two pairs of running shoes (one road, one trail) are waiting neatly side-by-side in the hall.

Another mistake I've made before – turning up for an ultra without proper shoes. The previous year I ran all 62 miles in tatty, long-since retired trainers with flapping soles and zero cushioning. For a moment I consider continuing to Winchester and trying to borrow some trainers at the start, or even running barefoot – anything but return to the scenes of mayhem I've surely left behind me.

I do return home of course, and in the five minutes I've been gone, Caroline has somehow calmed the dog and put all three kids back to bed. As well as tidied away my breakfast and helpfully left all the shoes outside the front door so I don't have to come back in. If it was the other way round, I'd probably have stuck on a film for us all.

The only mandatory kit I'm lacking is a water bottle so I stop at Winchester services and buy some mineral water. Then it's straight to registration and kit check. They randomly ask to see two items from the extensive list and I'm thrilled when water bottle is one of them. Feels like a little win, which is much needed to help assuage my pre-race nerves.

The feeling of apprehension borders on dread as I look around at my 500 fellow runners. They all look annoyingly fit and well prepared. I'm reminded of something I once heard from an ultra-running veteran. He says in general life, he walks around feeling fit and lean like Mo Farah, but on the start line of a 100-miler he feels like a sumo wrestler.

I start a few tentative conversations in the dawn light but soon think better of it. Everyone I speak to has successfully completed at least one of these in the past, and three people cheerfully tell me they've run dozens. Where are the hapless plonkers like me who forget their shoes and are beginning to feel ill from over-eating?

I take a seat on the some nearby steps and nervously await the briefing. The more I think about it – I can't help myself – the more convinced I am that I probably won't finish. I've done as much training as can, juggling several jobs and three separate school runs. I've only managed one long run since my last road marathon, and that was barely 35 miles. What on earth possessed me to think I could run 100? A hundred hilly miles – in one go? And do it inside a time limit? Another fine mess....

I'm looking down at my feet, wondering whether to swap my road runners for trail shoes, when suddenly a pair of jeans dominates my view. Above them, a fleece jacket – and a friendly face. It's Tim, a pal I made last summer during my only previous ultra, the 62-mile

Race to the Stones. We met around halfway through that glorious run between the Chiltern Hills and Avebury stone circle. We subsequently ran the rest of the race together, finished it together and kept in touch. Quite near the end, we'd passed someone using the race as her final training run before stepping up from 100km to the full 100 miles. We'd both decided, Tim and I, 55-odd miles into our first ultra, that our present labours were more than enough to be going on with – and vowed never *ever* to be so stupid as to attempt to run any further. Let the 100-mile brigade keep their commemorative belt buckles, we pronounced, and swore not to join their number under any circumstances.

The very next day, due to a calamitous diary clash, I'd driven to Derby and raced Jenson Button's sprint triathlon: the swim was surprisingly lovely, I was second out of the water, but the bike was feeble, and the run truly horrific. But even after that, and less than 24 hours after swearing never to consider a 100-miler, Tim and I had started texting each other about the possibility.

It gets you that way, this sport.

It also makes you the kind of friend who'll haul himself out of bed ridiculously early on a Saturday morning just because he lives quite close to the start and thinks you might need some moral support. Tim's arrival, just as I'm succumbing to self-doubt, is ridiculously welcome. I'm so grateful I nearly hug him. Then I do hug him. Several times. (Sorry, Tim.)

We giggle our way through the pre-race briefing (sorry James), then all of a sudden, the sound of a hooter and time to start running. My legs feel fresh and bouncy as they always do when I've not run on them for a few days. It's only a few weeks after they were at their best ever during the London Marathon – and they keep wanting me to speed up. I fervently hope the legs will continue to feel this good later this morning. And this afternoon. And evening. And overnight. Right now, if I was only running a flat marathon (as opposed to four hilly marathons back to back), I'd fancy my chances of a PB.

As it happens, I'm running at the only pace I can – everybody else's – until the path widens and the runners thin. I wait in a (mostly) orderly queue to climb over a stile and look to see who's texting me a photograph so early in the weekend.

It's Tim. He took the photo minutes earlier as I ran past him in the field – and as I look at the screen it's my own face grinning nervously back at me. The caption reads: 'Almost there! Just 99.75 miles to go...'.

I laugh, vault the stile, and speed up. My legs feel epic.

I start conversations with fellow runners but keep finding I'm desperate to run quicker than they are. The challenge of the many miles ahead makes me feel alive. I'm free, happy and fast. And then I meet somebody who makes me appreciate just how slow I really am.

Debbie Martin-Consani has represented GB in 100km and 24-hour endurance races. She once knocked a cool two-and-a-half hours off the previous record in the Lakeland 100-mile race whilst finishing second. She rectified that a year later by winning and when I meet her she's fresh from victory and a new course record in the SDW100's lesser-known sister, the North Downs Way 100. She accomplishes all this whilst working in a full-time job and raising a family. She's also really friendly.

I find I'm going at about the same pace as Debbie, which is ace, because I get to chat to her. Debbie knows she's currently third woman, though she doesn't seem remotely worried about not winning. Her forte, she tells me, is maintaining a relatively even pace throughout the 100 miles while all around her tire. It's a horrendously difficult trick to pull off.

'Would you take second place and a decent time?' I ask her. The reply is quiet and humble, but steely: 'No.'

I soon learn what it takes to become an elite ultra-runner. The levels of dedication. Debbie lives in Glasgow where she's a marketing manager, but she's recce-d every inch of the South Downs Way. That's a lot of weekend motorway miles and many nights in the campervan, all to make sure there are no surprises on race day. By contrast, despite the fact that we frequently visit my lovely in-laws who live within a mile or two of the famous footpath, the best I've managed is a 12-mile jog one January afternoon before some fog descended and I panicked. All sorts of nightmare scenarios went through my mind that day as I fretted about getting lost in the mist.

This morning by contrast, the weather's glorious, the sky is California blue and all around are grand, green hills – some have already been conquered, others still need vanquishing. Legs still sprightly 18 miles in, and I'm relishing every step.

I run with Debbie for most of the way between Aid Station One (nine miles in) and Two (at mile 23). Time enough for her to be very generous with advice for a newbie like me. 'You won't really know what sort of race you'll have until the final 20 miles or so,' she tells me. Gulp! 80 miles is 18 further than I've ever run before, and if I'm honest, I was rather hoping that by mile 80, I'd be on the home stretch, both mentally and physically. Tough to learn that runners can feel strong for fully 80% of a race like this, only to struggle so badly that they're forced to pull out. Mentally I reset the halfway mark to 75 miles, just like mile 20 is subliminally midway through a marathon.

Debbie also has time to eulogise about a race called the Spartathlon, which she completed the previous summer. This is the first I've heard of it, and a seed is sown. As a Greek, I love the idea of running in Greece – I *still* haven't managed to organise the diary well enough to allow me to run the Athens Classic Marathon, which finishes in the magnificent, all-marble, monumental Panathenaic Stadium, but every November I kick myself for not making the time; next year, definitely.

Even an experienced ultra-runner like Debbie becomes animated when describing the Spartathlon. I learn that the arrival of the competitors in Sparta is nothing short of epic, with kids running victoriously through the town with the splendid few who make it within the allotted time. There's no finishing line, just a statue of the Spartan warrior-king Leonidas, made famous by the film *300*. Exhausted runners simply touch or kiss the statue and they're done. It was a rare rainy day in

Greece when Debbie ran the race and finished fifth. As a Scot, she was apparently one of the few competitors smiling, enjoying the appalling weather – generally feeling right at home.

I learn too about the tribulations of 24-hour running. My new friend has represented Great Britain several times in endurance championships and is remarkably lucid and clear-headed about a race that exists, it seems, to do just the opposite and mess with your mind. This is from her blog:

It's a ridiculous concept, yet intriguing and challenging. On paper, it's simple. See how far you can run in 24 hours. Super slow running on mostly flat and looped courses, with copious amounts of support and no navigation or mandatory kit required. But those who have ventured into the crazy world of 24-hour running know that it's an emotionally, mentally and physically challenging journey.

There is no finish line so you can't DNF. There are no checkpoints to tick off and there's nothing to strive towards. It's you against the clock. A clock that you'll be convinced doesn't move.

Many great athletes can run 100 or 150 miles in a race, but don't have the head for 24-hour running. Without sections or a finish line it's hard to keep going. The clock keeps ticking regardless of what pace you're doing. Bravado doesn't even see you through 12 hours.

Debbie's also got 10 top tips for 24-hour races. Not, she says, because she's an expert but because she's made so many mistakes. 'I've never had a 24-hour go right, but some have been less catastrophic than others.' On one occasion, whilst visiting a portaloo at night, she was gingerly using her arms to lower herself onto the seat when she realised that the previous occupant had missed the pan – leaving Debbie to run the rest of the race with her hands covered in human excrement.

So, what's it like running as far as possible in a given time, rather than running a set distance as fast as possible? In cycling they have the fabled Hour – how far can you pedal in 60 minutes? It's widely considered to be the most brutal event in competitive cycling. Even the legendary Eddy Merckx, with his prodigious ability to tolerate suffering, was almost broken by the effort. 'This hour,' he said, 'was the longest of my life. The Hour demands a total effort, permanent and intense. I will never try it again.' And he didn't. So that's the greatest cyclist of all time after cycling as far as he could in one hour. How about running as far as you can in 24? Here are Debbie Martin-Consani's Top 10 Tips for 24-hour racing. I've got to admit I'm tempted to give it a shot.

1   Don't count the laps. You'll go nuts. If possible try to avoid looking at the clock too. It doesn't actually move.

2   Focus on lap splits or one hour at a time. Or split the race into day-night-day sections. If you're lucky, your race might turn direction every few hours, which will blow your mind!

3   Make the challenge to run for 24 hours – with the goal distance being secondary. You will be torn between the drive to stay on your feet and the devil on your shoulder screaming at you to stop. Once you start drifting from your target goal, the devil will win.

4   Be prepared to reassess your goals. Possibly about 17 times.

5   When you get to eight hours you will probably want to die. That's normal. Embrace the darkness: the night-time is always my favourite as I enjoy the cooler temperatures, the peace and the fact that a big chunk of the field is now off the course. Usually due to bad pacing.

6   Races are won and lost in the last four hours, so don't worry if someone is running Yiannis Kouros ('Running God') pace for the first few hours. The make-up of the race completely changes. Japan's Yoshihiko Ishikawa, who won the 2017 World Championships in Belfast with 267km, was in 90th position. 90th! That's what you call moving through the field.

7   Things happen in 24 hours that don't happen in other ultras. Feet take a real battering. You will be using the same muscles to

the point of destruction. And nausea will be your friend. You will probably witness more peeing, farting and spewing than you can imagine.

8   Treat yourself: keep your iPod for desperate stages, have a walking break on the hour, save the pee stop for the next hour. Trust me, it's the best seat in the house. It's little things that make a big difference.

9   Smile and be polite to crew/volunteers. It forces your mind to stay positive.

10 You have to really want it. If you don't, you'll find an excuse.

There's no question that Debbie really wants it, both the race win here and ultra-running success generally. But why did she decide to start running long?

It was a bit of an accident really. It was 2007 and I was looking for my next race online. I stumbled on the Devil o' the Highlands, which takes in the last 43 miles of the West Highland Way. I remember sending my husband an email with the subject line: *We've run marathons, how hard can it be?* In reality, it was very hard and I was broken at the end. The route goes through Glen Coe, and I was woefully unprepared for the rocky paths and the hills. But I loved it and I was hooked, despite saying it was going to be my one and only ultra. I signed up for the full West Highland Way Race the year after and the rest is history.

'What do you love about it?'

Mainly that the possibilities are endless. Unlike traditional road race distances, there are always new ways to challenge yourself, explore new places and try new distances and races. I love the camaraderie between ultra-runners, but I also love the adrenaline and tactics of racing ultra-distances. It's not always about racing fast, it's about racing smart. The latter suits me, because I don't have the raw speed to compete well in shorter races, but I take great joy (and a few scalps) in pacing well. I've also had the opportunity to run on the GB team for five years, which has been an amazing experience. Ultra-racing takes me on some amazing journeys, often seeing places in one go. Like Transgrancanaria, which runs along the spine of the island, from Athens to Sparta in Spartathlon, or 200 miles in the Italian Alps in Tor des Géants.

Debbie hasn't noticed that she's doing most of the talking whilst I'm happily firing questions at her and enjoying a breather while she answers. Or perhaps she has noticed, and simply doesn't mind. Either way, I try to keep the questions open so her answers (and my rest periods) will be longer. Plus, how often do you get the chance to chat to the race winner mid-race?

'Your husband Marco is also a GB ultra-runner. How do you juggle family and training when both parents work and run silly distances?!'

My motto is: I don't find the time, I make the time. I say this to anyone who says they don't have time to exercise. Taking into account the working day, a commute and a good night's sleep, the average person has approximately 60 hours of free time a week. I fit in the miles around work, family and an ultra-running husband by running to and from work, doing speed sessions at lunchtime and getting out early at the weekend. I don't really get the opportunity to enjoy nights out, lie-ins, relaxing weekends or even wait for the rain to stop. But that suits me as running is more important. I organise my training week – knowing exactly when I'm going to run – and I stick to it. If you want something, you will find a way.

'Did you meet Marco while running?'

Yes, we met at our local running club in Glasgow, Garscube Harriers. We both joined around the same time in 2005. I had run two London Marathons so I convinced Marco to run a marathon, saying he wasn't a real runner until he'd run 26.2 miles. I'm not sure of the logic behind that, because now I know 10Ks and half marathons are way harder than running long distances.

'What's it like to have started something brilliant like Marcothon, where people sign up to run a minimum of three miles or 25 minutes every day during December?'

It's quite overwhelming how quickly something which started from a conversation in our living room led to thousands of people all over the world running on Christmas Day. For no reason or reward whatsoever. The vast majority of people who 'sign up' don't know either of us. Some people even think it's a memorial event! The Marcothon started in 2009, but I don't think it had an official name that year. Our son Cairn was born in early 2009 and Marco was looking for a way to deal with injuries and motivation and get back into some consistent training. He decided to run every day in November, with his rules being a minimum of three miles or 25 minutes. I decided to follow suit in December and posted on my blog to see if anyone wanted to join me. I think about 50 people may have started, mostly friends and local runners. The year after I put it on Facebook and 500 joined. Now we're up to over 5,000 and it grows every year.

Of course it would be easier to run the event in the summer, but December is what makes it so unique. People lack motivation and time, so this gets people out of the door and maintaining fitness. And burning off a few Christmas lunches and hangovers. There are even people who start running from scratch just to complete this. The social media support is so amazing that nobody dares not to run because it's raining or windy. There's a big emphasis on it being a personal goal and it's just for fun. There's no focus on speed and no need to document or prove anything, it's just about getting outside when a night on the sofa eating mince pies may be way more appealing.

Debbie and I arrive together at the aid station in Queen Elizabeth Country Park. Marco and Cairn, her husband and son, are waiting with arms outstretched – not offering hugs and kisses but pre-assigned hydration and sustenance.

I don't really see or understand what happens next, it's too quick, too well-drilled – reminding me actually of a Formula One pit stop. You know what's taking place but it's so slick, every movement so well-rehearsed, that it just seems like a blur and suddenly it's all over.

One second Debbie and I are chatting amiably, the next I'm glancing down at the volunteers' table next to where the Consanis are standing, picking up a peanut butter and jam wrap, and she's *disappeared*. Completely disappeared. Presumably onwards up a hill, munching on the food she's just been given. Of all the surprises that assail the senses in my first 100-mile race, this is probably the most startling. That in a race which will take 17 hours at least, refuelling stops are practised – to avoid losing precious seconds. It makes sense of course. Like they say in British Cycling, it's the 'aggregation of marginal gains': if you improve everything by even 1%, then those small gains will add up to a remarkable improvement.

Predictably, as I chomp down on the heavenly wrap (I may have already mentioned, peanut butter and jam being undeniably the finest sandwich filling known to mankind: I think we may have peaked, as a species, when we discovered it), that's the last I see of the woman known in these circles as Ultra-Run-DMC. She does go on to win the women's race – easily – and finishes sixth overall.

I linger for much longer at the aid station, enjoying conversations with the ever-wonderful volunteers and especially enjoying the food. Despite my gargantuan breakfast, I'm already starving. I stand around near the table, chatting, eating, generally blissfully unaware of anything remotely resembling the concept of a race, or even a mild hurry. I'm enjoying myself and the only real target I've set myself for today is to finish inside the 24-hour mark. You get a different belt buckle if you're any longer, and I definitely want the one that says *100 Miles – One Day*. (The other reads *100 Miles – Finisher*, which may look cooler to the untrained eye, but I'd know.)

Eventually one of the volunteers, a seasoned, currently injured, ultra-runner, suggests I may want to be on my way, and schools me in aid station best practice before I go. This involves calling out your race number as you arrive and asking for containers to be refilled with your choice of water, squash or sports drink. While that happens, you grab as much food as you can carry from the table. One of the added motivations to run quickly is that fewer grubby hands have been at the food before you. As soon as the newly refilled water bottles are returned, you set off, eating the food as you go. This is why aid stations – certainly in the best-organised ultras – tend to be located at the bottom of lengthy hills, so you can briskly walk up whilst eating without losing too much time (as you'd be unlikely to run the hills anyway).

I start up the hill at a steady march, still waiting for the first sign of any fatigue or leg-related aches and pains. Indeed any bodily complaint at all. This is all going suspiciously well. I think back to my only previous ultra and realise I'm almost certainly in for a nasty surprise further down the South Downs Way. I'd begun Race to the Stones similarly issue-free, but I shudder as I remember the pain from 50 miles onwards. Every footfall seemed to judder through my quad muscles like a lorry. I'd been running with Tim (who saw me off at the start today) and he struggled too. I vividly remember why we vowed never to attempt a 100-miler: if it's this bad now, we reasoned, how much worse would it become after another half-marathon? And after another one again – at 85 miles? How about after running 95 miles, with fully five miles still to run?

There's nobody about to chat to as I pass full marathon distance, and all of a sudden I feel a little jangle of nerves. A shiver of fear despite the heat of the day. Earning the belt buckle is, I fear, going to sting.

Trying to remain positive I think back to everything that I *loved* about the 100km on the Ridgeway. It's Britain's oldest footpath, so you're following in the footsteps of Vikings, Romans, kings and dragons. From a field just north of High Wycombe to an ancient stone circle just south of Swindon, the path meanders through some truly majestic countryside. Past ancient forts and prehistoric hill figures, through verdant cornfields, sun-dappled woods and idyllic villages complete with wickedly inviting riverside pubs. The scenery can't help but give tiring legs a lift. And even though it may be a cliché, I discovered that an ultra is a chance to find out some stuff about yourself. That day I realised – in the words of the organisers, Threshold Sports – that 'More Is In Me'.

The memories help to lighten my mood considerably. The South Downs are equally stunning today, the sun is shining, and I'm running. Nothing to worry about except reaching Eastbourne. Literally all I need to do today is keep going. Just me and the trail. It's liberating.

11. eastbourne

James Elson is the man who runs the SDW100. We've spoken a few times on the phone in the week or two leading up to the race, I see him briefly at several points along the way, call him when I contrive to get lost, and meet him properly at the finish. He's another excellent human being; this sport seems to breed them. He organises eight major ultra-races every year, runs a kit and equipment shop, records a weekly podcast, coaches keen amateurs and competes for GB. But when I ask him for one story that defines his ultra-running career, he doesn't even feature in it.

For me it's just about the people crossing our finishing line. Probably the most emotional finish we had was two ladies who were running on behalf of a children's charity down in Dorset. They look after children who've lost their parents to cancer. These kids have got nobody, they're being cared for by these wonderful people, and they all came down to the track to see these two ladies finish.

You just can't even begin to fathom the sort of depth of emotion that's going on for the runners, for the kids, and for the staff, everybody there. And that is an amazing thing. On the selfish side, you're giving runners the opportunity to experience something incredible, but when it goes beyond that to reaching out to friends and family and literally changing people's lives, that means a great deal and it's definitely the most fulfilling part of what we do. The part that makes it all worthwhile.

Last week we had a guy running after the loss of his son, in his memory, and then he went straight on to hang his finisher buckle on his son's grave. Where do you begin with that stuff? There are also many stories of triumph, which are wonderful – but perhaps the sadder tales have greater depth of meaning. Of course I've felt great achievement at some of the things I've done myself too, but that is so purely selfish that I think it's very short-lived in relation to the other things, if that makes sense.

He's getting emotional even as he speaks. You can tell he feels it. To give him a chance to recover his composure as much as anything, I ask a prosaic question about how and why he went from competing in 100-mile races to organising them. A prosaic question, with an enlightening answer.

I went to the US to do a couple of 100-milers to qualify for Badwater. So for me it was a means to an end at first. But then I realised that here in the UK, we were missing that scene. We didn't have many 100-milers and those we did have were unmarked, had little support and we were asking people to orienteer or navigate for the distance. I felt that was adding a component that didn't necessarily need to be part of it. Of course navigating, map reading, it's a hugely alluring part of many UK challenges, for example the Dragon's Back Race. It's part of UK ultra-running heritage. But I felt we didn't have a gateway option for new people who wanted to run the distance but couldn't get down and recce the course or couldn't afford to. I thought they should be able to race on an equal footing, since the first time you want to focus on one thing, and that's putting one foot in front of the other, rather than getting lost or trying to navigate through the night. I wanted to strip away a lot of the additional components and do what I had enjoyed very much in the US. Being able to run the race without having to worry about those other things.

Then I looked at our big national trails that are wonderful institutions. There weren't any races on them, and that didn't seem right. I knew they'd be popular. So I decided to bring a very American format over to the UK. That hasn't been everybody's cup of tea. I mean I'm sure there are a lot of people who think, 'Why the hell are you marking a national trail? They're already safely way-marked.' But for the majority of runners, that's a massive benefit. It takes a lot of guesswork out of the equation and allows you to focus on enjoying your run, not spending half the time looking at the map.

So, I think it's been well received, but the amount of work that goes into our races is huge. Marking a full 100 miles! So we made a rod for our own back in a way.

The original 100-mile footrace started life as a horserace. In the 1950s, five pioneers wanted to know whether horses could still cover 100 miles in one day, and rode the Western States Trail from the post office in Tahoe City to Auburn, California – thus founding the annual Western States Trail Ride, or Tevis Cup. Then in 1974, a rider called Gordy Ainsleigh's horse went lame so he decided to see if he could complete the course on foot. He could. Others followed suit and three years later the first official Western States Endurance Run was born. There were 14 men who started that first race; three finished. These days the race has an almost mythical status among ultra-runners. James based the SDW100 entirely on Western States.

As soon as you get into the 100-mile scene, Western States comes onto your horizon. You hear about it everywhere because it was the first one, when Gordy decided he was going to run instead of ride. Something special was born. And in many ways Western States is the perfect template for our sport. The trail is varied, and there are really distinctive sections. There are some truly great vistas, it's fairly remote, and they don't have a lot of runners. But they do have a lot of volunteers, a lot of support for a relatively small group of people.

It's a very iconic start in Squaw Valley. And as for the finish in Auburn on the track… it's just a high-school running track, it shouldn't be the great arena of ultra-running, but it is. Because for 40 years, Western States has finished on that high-school track.

And I think running around the track is a genius touch. Just to have that special finish to a race. I mean some people think, 'Why the hell do I want to run around this track after I've run this whole trail?' But it's almost like a two-minute celebration of everything up to that point. You get a few minutes to reflect upon what it is you've done. Within sight of the finish line, you can really enjoy it.

And yeah, the belt buckle thing. It's come from the horse-riding heritage obviously. But that's the idea I wanted to bring to the UK. People weren't giving belt buckles out before we started at the South Downs 100. It helps to separate out the 100-mile distance from anything less. It is something that is synonymous with that distance.

That belt buckle is something I'm determined to earn. I reach another aid station and resolve to spend much less time chatting and eating. This is easier said than done as the volunteers are all so friendly and welcoming, and the food so enticing. But much as I want to stand around and chew the fat (and the food), I force myself to do as I've been taught, grab some sustenance and eat it on the hoof.

Hiking up a lengthy hill, I start talking to a fellow runner called Sam Robson. He has impressive sideburns and an equally impressive pedigree. He once finished second in this race, and tries to complete four or five ultras every year. I wonder how on earth he has time and, as a fellow family man, how he gets permission frankly. He seems to be well known and well liked by everyone we meet along the way.

One of the first races he tells me about is the Spartathlon. Sam was first British finisher in 2014, and like Debbie Martin-Consani, was blown away by the whole experience. Especially the finish in Sparta. I'm beginning to feel the draw of the Peloponnese, even though I'm still 50 miles from Eastbourne.

Sam also recounts the story of the so-called 'Ball of String' race organised by a friend of his. You turn up at an appointed time and place, with absolutely no idea how far you'll be running. Just before the start, an envelope is selected at random, one of three, and that determines the race route. But only for the organiser. Still competitors are none the wiser; the race could be shorter than 10 miles, or longer than 100. You're simply told to run to a certain place, which is either the end or the next stepping-stone on the adventure – you find out when you get there.

Eventually, some 24 hours later, Sam was the last man standing. He arrived at a checkpoint utterly exhausted, drained, in urgent need of sleep. Despite the protestations of the race director, he passed out in the back seat of a car. Little did Sam know he was actually at the penultimate checkpoint, a mere three miles from the finish. What a pity if he chose to abandon here. Ten minutes later, to relief all round, he woke up feeling refreshed and completed the race.

He's equally determined to finish this one, having been forced to pull out 93 miles into last year's edition. It shocks me, as we approach the major checkpoint at mile 54, that pulling out so late is even an option for someone so experienced. I'd assumed you could crawl the final few miles if necessary.

We run past a wedding party outside a church in the pretty village of Washington, and arrive at the biggest aid station. It's in a village hall, there's hot food and an inside toilet, crews mill about waiting for the runners they're supporting, and any drop bags from the start have been delivered here too. It's tempting, having run 54 hilly miles, to have a proper break, a nice sit down, perhaps change my shirt and socks, even have a power nap. However, I know it'll be immeasurably harder to get going again if I do. So after a quick visit to the loo I head straight back through the door, up the hill and past the joyful bride and groom who are now smiling enthusiastically for photographs.

Sam and I end up running together for the next 20-odd miles, chatting all the way. At one point I'm boosted by some surprise support from my ace brother- and sister-in-law bringing their brilliant boys all the way to the top of Devil's Dyke (they live near the bottom) to cheer me along.

My legs are tiring, but not dramatically, and otherwise I feel terrific. I'm still running with a permanent smile on my face. Sam fancies my chances from here on in, but remembering what Debbie told me about the halfway point being 75 miles, I'm not counting any chickens.

Occasionally we pass other runners, some of whom have pacers with them, and Sam seems to know them all. Near the top of a long hill 68 miles in, we see a competitor walking slowly back towards us.

'Are you OK, mate?'

'Not good, going to have to bail.'

'What's up?'

'Weeing blood. Lots of it.'

That sounds worryingly serious to me, but Sam pulls a face as if it's relatively normal.

'Are you sure it's bad enough to pull out?'

'Definitely.'

It turns out this is an experienced ultra-runner, and he knows his limits of what's normal in this sphere. Blood in the urine during (or after) a long run is usually caused when the walls of your empty bladder rub together. Nothing to be alarmed about, it's kind of a rite of passage. However, if the wee is particularly dark and red, it could mean a bigger issue involving the kidneys, infections or renal shutdown.

Instinctively Sam and I turn to walk back to the nearest aid station with the ailing runner. Just seems like the right thing to do. It's about a mile away at the bottom of the hill. Our new friend is having none of it.

'Seriously guys, thank you, but I can manage.'

'Don't be silly, we're happy to help.'

'No I mean it. Thanks but no thanks.'

'Really mate, don't worry about it. We're coming with you just in case.'

'I *insist* you don't.'

It's said with such feeling that we know he means it. He then adds, rather wonderfully:

'But just so you know, you're the fourth and fifth runners I've seen since I turned back. And every single one of you has tried to walk me to the aid station. You've all been willing to sacrifice time and add miles.'

This exchange has stayed with me. I just love the fact that ultra-runners are the sort of people who think nothing of sabotaging their own race to help someone in trouble. I especially like the fact that I seem to have become that sort of person. Another reason to fall for this sport.

Sam and I run on together but soon his stomach begins to grumble. Trust me, a tummy issue when you've been running for 70 miles is like no tummy issue you've ever experienced. Difficult to ignore, often impossible to run through. Sam decides to take 15 minutes at the next aid station, and demands that I carry on without him. I'm sorry to leave Sam sitting bent double in a chair, and thankful that my own stomach seems to be behaving itself. My legs are truly worn out but I still feel generally well and happy. Less than a marathon to go.

It takes a special kind of idiot to get lost on the South Downs Way. In addition to all the official way markings, the race organisers have tied red and white-striped tape to trees, posts etc. every 20 or 30 yards. I catch a small group ahead of me, two competitors and a pacer, and run with them for a while. It dawns on me that I'm travelling a little better so I decide to press on. But in that particular stretch, there are lots of gates and stiles. Several times, I find myself gaining a few dozen yards, only to stand and wait whilst holding open a gate. I do consider leaving the gates to close behind me, but I'm not quite far enough ahead for that not to be a bit rude.

A long, grassy, gate-free descent and I'm away. It's getting dark now and I consider stopping to retrieve my head torch from my rucksack. But I'm making good progress and the next aid station isn't far. Seems a shame to stop now. So I plough on, missing the red and white tape that would have been obvious in the light of a torch, and turning left along a road instead of crossing straight over it.

A mile or so later, I realise I've not seen any tape for ages. I retrace my steps, increasingly agitated. The next aid station is in the village of Southease and I follow a road sign into the village centre. It's properly dark now and I'm belatedly wearing the torch, but I can't find the aid station anywhere. I knock at a cottage door and ask whether I'm still on the South Downs Way. The woman who answers says she thinks so. I run back to the road crossing hoping to see some tape, and then back through the village again.

Only call the race director in an emergency, it says in the notes. Does this count as an emergency? Not even close, but I phone James anyway.

'I'm really sorry to be calling, James. I'm lost in Southease. Could you possibly let me know where the aid station is please?'

James to his credit manages to sound calm and reassuring when he has every right to hang up on me. Five minutes and a level crossing later, I arrive at the 84-mile checkpoint and see two friendly faces at once. First my wife, who's put the kids to bed and driven here to surprise me. And standing next to her, having recovered from his stomach issues and overtaken me whilst I was lost on the wrong path, is Sam.

I get quite tearful when I see my wife and/or kids during a properly long run. The physical trauma you're putting yourself through seems to strip away all the usual layers and what's left is a blubbing mess. All that pain, all those hours on your feet, you're simultaneously strong, immersed in the moment, but also naked, fragile. I try to hold it together and fail magnificently. I'm surreptitiously wiping my eyes as Sam and I set off to tackle the 16 remaining miles.

We've been running together for so long we're running out of conversation. We resort to listing our favourite films and music, which whiles away another few miles to the penultimate aid station. Quick pause here for a cup of tea, and straight through the final checkpoint without stopping.

We climb one final hill and soon after we reach the top, the route turns off the Downs down a rutted, chalky path. Sam claims you can fly down this, 6-minute-mile-ing, even at the end of an ultra, but I'm not so sure. It's narrow, twisty, tree roots everywhere. They call it Death Alley. We're discharged from the path into the northern suburbs of Eastbourne. At this point there's less than two miles left to run, all on flat tarmac. I'd been looking forward to these final miles as a sort of 'free hit'. My legs have other ideas. I've already run more than 100 miles at this stage (because of the extra three I managed whilst lost) and my legs are suddenly rebelling.

This morning, it seems my subconscious mind sent a message to the legs demanding that they propel me 100 miles. Now they've accomplished it, the legs want out. These easy miles I'd been anticipating are proving to be the hardest of the entire race. It's taking every scintilla of willpower to keep running, and my speed is down to a shuffle.

Sam, bless him, stays with me. Eventually we reach the running track. Those final 400 metres are utterly thrilling. Like James says, they're a celebration of everything that's gone before. And completing your first 100-miler, that feeling, it's solid gold.

I'm surprised to learn that we finished joint 23rd in 19 hours or so. Much quicker than I'd dared hope for. But it's a strangely humbling feeling as I'm presented with my *100 Miles – One Day* belt buckle. It feels like so many others deserve it at least as much as I do. The volunteers manning the aid stations so ably and graciously; the organisers; Tim, Dani and my gorgeous nephews who braved the rain to say hello at Devil's Dyke; Sam, Debbie and the others who ran with me; and of course Caroline, who's here hugging me on the track and who's helped with so much more.

There's no euphoria after crossing the line. It's much better than that. A deep contentment rises from the pit of your stomach and seems to settle in. I haven't experienced this in shorter races, even the 62-miler. That race seemed to hurt more, but didn't have this finish line euphoria. Or perhaps it hurt the same and I'm just used to that trashed feeling in the front of your thighs. Either way, running 100 miles seems somehow to complete the circle. James is at the finish too; I ask him why he thinks running 100 miles is so special.

I think it's several things. To be totally honest, I think the number is a big part of it. You know in Europe it's 161 kilometres but to us in the UK, it's simply a huge, round number. When you say it, when you think about it – it's sort of mind blowing. It seems about as hard and as far as it's ever going to get without becoming silly or requiring a lot of sleep to get through it.

125

Also I think there's a thrill to it. This is going to take you through the night, pretty much guaranteed. It's so much more substantial than even 100 kilometres. You know the old ultra-running adage, '100 miles is like three 50 milers'. I think that's very true. It's the whole adventure of being up all night, running under a head-lamp for many of the hours that you wouldn't get in shorter distances.

Plus the fact that something is probably going to go fairly badly wrong at some point, and you have to solve that and keep going. So the sense of achievement is that much greater.

Anything up to say 10 or 12 hours, I think a lot of people can almost get by on fumes. When you go beyond that you're asking something of your body. You're going to have to take it to a place it would never ordinarily go. You're going to have to do things nutritionally that you've not done before.

Maybe one day we can dream that people will be lining the streets for the runners coming in through Eastbourne.

It's clear James loves organising the race as much as I've just enjoyed running it. He's been known to secretly compete in his own events too, and even win them. He'll give the race briefing as normal, then strip to reveal a running kit and a race number, and calmly charge off with everybody else.

His company, Centurion Running, organises eight events every year, four 100-milers and four 50s. But Centurion as a whole sustains one person, James, and it requires a coaching business, a retail business, and an events business to do it. But all his events sell out and he could clearly make life more comfortable simply by hiking up his prices, or opening up the marquee events to many more people. There's a waiting list just to volunteer for the SDW100.

We love it, you know? We just love being with everybody over those weekends. And long may that continue. We don't look for massive numbers. The South Downs 100, the easy thing would have been to open it up and make it bigger and bigger, 500 entrants, 800, 1,000. There are some ultras in the UK which are now that big. We're full at 300. If we increased the numbers like that, then we'd completely destroy the ethos of our events.

We want it to be like Western States where you show up, you're one of a small number of people who all have names. You're not just a number on a piece of paper. You get to experience the race, interact with the volunteers, in a very personal way. Also to have a lot of time to yourself on the trail, not be one of a huge number of people processed through to the finish. So we've capped it, we've held back. And we will continue to do that.

I never ever want a runner to cross the finish line at one of our events and feel like they've been ripped off. I have heard that before, runners use those exact words. If you come away from an event feeling that, the organisers probably got something badly wrong.

We try and make it about the sport and the people, not about the money. That's how you survive longer term, and have a sustainable event that enough people get to enjoy.

The more races that exist, the more volunteers are required to help them happen safely. We're digging very deep into a pool that isn't that deep, and it would be highly irresponsible for us to just keep digging and digging. What if the volunteer pool runs dry?

Worse, for these new starter events that are trying to get their feet off the ground, if there's no volunteers out there because they're all being sucked up by the established organisations, then they can't get started and we're losing the grass-roots of the sport. It's a sustainability issue on a number of levels.

More than anything, if you get into ultra-running to try and make money, you're just missing the point. This is about the lifestyle and the community. And ultimately it always comes back to the running, right? You've got to love the running part of it, and if you don't, then you're probably not going to be around in the sport for that long because it's just too hard otherwise.

12. sangas

It's pitch dark now in Greece. There's a long climb up a zigzag hill to get to the mountain base. The only light is coming from my head torch, a small, brilliant circle in front of me that bobs about as I move. The climb takes ages, never seems to end, and I love every moment.

Far below are two tiny pinpricks of light similarly weaving their way upwards. Fellow Spartathletes. They're the only visible clue that the race is happening. Elsewhere it's black, silent, Hellenic night. My laboured breathing reverberates around my head, keeping pace with my footsteps – two steps per breath.

I've been going a long time now and it amazes me, as it often does on a long run, that I've not been bored for a second. Yet I've been doing the exact same thing, running, for over 16 hours. I'm frequently asked: 'What on earth do you think about when you're out there for so long?' Well, as the writer Haruki Murakami notes in his book *What I Talk About When I Talk About Running*, that's almost beside the point. 'I just run,' he writes. 'I run in a void. Or maybe I should put it the other way: I run in order to acquire a void.'

Much has been made of running's ability to make you mindful. Absolutely in the present. And that's a wonderful, life-enhancing thing. However, running can also be mind*less*, and that's sometimes equally lovely. T.S. Eliot, the poet, described thinking as 'idea incubation'. To the inventor Alexander Graham Bell it was 'unconscious cerebration'. And the original American advertising executive James Webb Young says it's 'unconscious processing'. Whatever you want to call it, it's rather pleasant to be lost in your own random thoughts.

But now, something that's been lurking for several hours around the edge of my consciousness – a nagging, grating worry I've been trying to ignore – finally finds form. Pain in my right ankle. The one I injured during the Dragon's Back Race. Significant pain. Always worse when I'm going uphill, when my foot's bent forwards, like it is now.

I feel a momentary jolt of panic that the same injury will end another adventure prematurely. Then strangely, a calm certainty that I simply won't let it.

I decide to try something new, a theory I've heard. Instead of battling to disassociate myself from the problem, I concentrate deeply on the pain. I revel in it, dial down into it, allow it to fill my entire being. The theory goes that there's only a limited amount of information the nerves can send up to the brain before they become overloaded and give up. This is what somebody once told me over a pint. Nobody medical you understand, so please don't take it as fact. Or even as advisable. In fact this comes from another ultra-runner – and you know what we're like!

I keep concentrating on the ache in my ankle. It's liberating to be focusing on something I'd usually be trying to ignore. The pain swells, cascades, intensifies... and suddenly, dies.

Wow. This, I sense immediately, is a significant discovery, not simply for the purposes of reaching Sparta but for my future as a runner. I already have a somewhat laid back attitude to injuries: I reckon that for the most part the body will find a way to cope. If it's true that we were once persistence hunters who relied on running long distances for food, then surely we couldn't be stopped by the odd hip sprain or muscle tear. Our bodies would have found a way or we'd have starved. 'Stop moaning and get on with it' is basically the approach I adopt whenever I get a niggle, and it's largely worked. But then again, I've been pretty lucky of late.

By contrast, there's the physio's mantra of RICE, Rest Ice Compression Elevation, which doubtless aids healing. And when I first started running, I was frequently indebted to sports medicine professionals whenever something broke down, which was often. And the one time I tried to force an injured ankle around a five-day mountain race in Wales, I comprehensively failed.

However, this new concentrate-on-the-pain thing. Having made the ankle stop hurting, I almost want to try it on more injuries – if doing so wouldn't inherently mean more injuries. No, but hang on, how about my swollen left knee? That's been low-level aching most days since a badly judged triathlon four years ago. Worth a try.

I focus on the knee, and sure enough the inside of it gives a growl of displeasure. It's usually quite easy to ignore the hurty knee, but now I do the opposite and give it the freedom of my mind. I think about nothing but the pain in my knee. The stabbing sensation whenever I put weight on it, and the rude echo when I don't. The knee responds gleefully to its newfound attention, a toddler having a tantrum. It's hurting worse than at any time since the excruciating miles I ran on it whilst doing the initial damage. But just as I start to worry I'm doing the wrong thing and the knee could become a meaningful hurdle – once again the pain simply evaporates.

OK. Momentary pause for a public service announcement. Please don't try this at home. Or indeed, on the trail. I've not had a chance to experiment with it since, so can't entirely vouch for the fact that it works. All I know is that it did work on that Greek mountainside 99 miles from Athens.

Which is where we'll return now to find me arriving gratefully at the checkpoint at the bottom of the dark, rocky slopes. I'm offered soup by the wonderful volunteers but refuse. I want to get this done.

Yesterday, stupidly in retrospect, I opted to have my warm top delivered to the summit checkpoint, rather than the bottom like everybody else. My thinking was, I'll be working hard on the climb and won't need extra clothes to keep warm. That was just wrong. I'm freezing, shivering, teeth chattering despite the effort of climbing. The rocks are slippery in the intensifying rain. The wind is furious. This is where Pheidippides is said to have met Pan. The god called out to the messenger and asked why Athenians paid him little attention even though he'd helped them in the past. Pheidippides passed on the message and an altar to Pan was built at the Acropolis, where we began this race so many hours ago.

I've heard numerous stories of Spartathletes hallucinating on Mount Sangas. It's not hard to understand why. Exhaustion, hunger, burnout, depletion, darkness. Wind, rain and the light of your head torch casting strange shadows on the rocky mountainside. I bury myself in the effort and concentration of the ascent. Crib Goch it's not, but you definitely wouldn't want to slip and fall here.

Midway through the climb, my watch bleeps to tell me that I've hit 100 miles. It's taken me just over 17 hours, comfortably my fastest hundred. I'd enjoy the fact a little more if my watch didn't simultaneously beep to tell me it was almost out of battery. And if I wasn't so bloody cold. The extra T-shirt and makeshift bin bag jacket are clearly better than nothing, but they're not coming close to keeping out the icy wind and rain.

The volunteers at the top of the mountain are extraordinary, almost a different breed. It's blowing a gale up there, and by the time I arrive they've already been enduring the wind and rain for five solid hours. I complain loudly watching February football at Fulham's Craven Cottage, where a chill wind whips in from the River Thames and freezes you to your seat. My son frequently has to chisel me free at full time. The summit of Mount Sangas, 4,000 feet above sea level, beats it hands down for cold. And these volunteers don't get to go inside for a hot drink at half time. They climbed the mountain at 8pm. They'll stay up there all night until the checkpoint closes at 6am.

Right now, midway through their shift, they welcome me with huge smiles and shivering fingers. They insist on helping me into my jacket. I'm really quite moved by their uncomplaining, hardy kindness and give them all a sincere hug of thanks. They offer me tea but I really do have to get going. It's absolutely freezing up here.

The descent is slippery and treacherous. However, it's nice to be running again after such a long time hiking uphill. The quads have been given a bit of a breather for the past hour or two, and they appreciate it. This is further than I've ever run before, yet I'm still feeling OK. Whisper it quietly, but I'm increasingly confident of finishing. I'm fully five hours ahead of the cut-offs, and as people have been telling me all week – people rarely pull out after the top of the mountain.

Thoughts turn back to Pheidippides. As I canter down the slopes it's easy to believe I might be following in his actual footsteps. Harder to sustain that fantasy earlier in the race, obviously, running on tarmac past heavy industry with lorries roaring past. But here, on the bare mountain, I try to imagine what he'd have been thinking all those centuries ago. And indeed, what he'd have been thinking as he ran back to Athens the following day.

Because the thing is, Sparta said no.

Throughout the 153 miles and 36 hours of his heroic journey to the Peloponnese, Pheidippides would have been preparing what to say. The Spartans knew nothing of the impending Persian invasion, and the exhausted messenger would have had to persuade them to take up arms and join forces with the Athenians in what was bound to be a brutal battle with no guarantee of victory. And Sparta said no.

Or to be totally accurate, they said *not yet*. Their customs and beliefs forbade them from fighting unless it was a full moon – and that wasn't due for another week. The delay would prove fatal to the Athenian army marching to Marathon unless they knew about it. So Pheidippides had no choice but to turn around after the briefest of rests, and hurry back to Athens with the bad news. Which is exactly what he did, thereby completing a scarcely credible double Spartathlon.

A feat most recently achieved by a granny from Kent.

Mimi Anderson isn't your average British gran. She's known in ultra circles as Marvellous Mimi and her feats of endurance are legendary. She holds the world record for the fastest run from John O'Groats to Land's End. She was on course to annihilate the longstanding record for running across America – it stands at 69 days, Mimi was aiming for 53 – when a stress fracture derailed her. As well as the double Spartathlon, Mimi's done a double Badwater, a double Grand Union Canal Race, and broken the course record for the 352-mile Extreme Ultra Marathon in the Arctic. But she didn't always run. In fact she only started running to get better-looking legs.

Total and utter vanity. I was told that the best way to thinner legs was to take up running. So I just headed off to the gym and got myself onto the treadmill. Initially, I couldn't run for more than about five minutes without gasping for breath. But it was a case of just get to three miles. So I built it up on my treadmill until I could run for three miles.

Then a friend of mine just said, 'Look we're going to go and do a run outside, which is around 10 miles. So come and run with us.' It was seven miles further than I had ever run before, and the concept of running anywhere but a treadmill was an alien concept to me. But I just loved it. It was fantastic. And from there I did a few 10K races and half marathons. And then this friend of mine said, 'Right, here's our next race' and it was an article about the Marathon des Sables*. I remember it was in *The Times*, in their magazine. And there were lots of pictures, and you know, blisters and people suffering in the heat. And it was so far fetched from my world that I just thought, 'I've got to go and do that.'

Mimi suffered from an eating disorder for many years, the legacy of the abuse she suffered as a child at the hands of a cruel nanny. She's very candid when writing about it. But now, when she goes training or embarks on one of her epic adventures, she doesn't feel she's running away from anything.

Not any more. I don't think I ever felt that when I started running. Because I felt that I'd dealt with my demons by the time I took up running. So I think for me, rather than running away from something, it just gave a

---

* The Marathon des Sables, or MdS, is possibly the most famous ultra in the world. It's well marketed anyway as it's the only one many people have heard of. Six days and 120 miles over the Moroccan Sahara desert. It was once high on my to-do list, but it's slipped down a little.

sense of freedom actually. It was time away from the children, away from my husband – in the nicest possible way. And just time to myself. It was me time.

For me again, running is all about seeing different parts of the world, so you know a lot of the races I've done, like the Arctic, I've chosen because of the distance, and also because of the location. And because my husband Tim's never going to take me there on holiday. I have to go to run there. But I think also, it's just part of my personality. How far can I push myself? Am I capable of running 153 miles, 300 miles, 1,000 miles? Can I do it? So I think it's testing myself the whole time. Going out there, it's just the whole package. It's the challenge. I like being out there and I like the planning.

I don't go into great details. I'm not a great one for elevation and pace and all that jazz because you can set yourself a pace and quite frankly you don't always keep to it. So I like to go out there and enjoy the moment. I mean yes, I'm racing, but actually doing the best I can. If I can't get a certain pace, well that doesn't matter. You can wake up in the morning and be in a foul mood…. You can put everything into little cubby holes and come back and the day starts afresh, you know. So yeah, it's testing myself more than anything else, really.

I'm keen to find out what it's like to run across a country. Her first attempt to run from Land's End to John O'Groats ended prematurely through injury. Second time around (going the other way, north to south) she succeeded in breaking the previous record – by 36 minutes. That's 13 days of constant running, up at 4:30 am, taking only short breaks for food and sleep, and all with the pressure of the record hanging over her every step.

It's hard. Very hard. Mentally as much as anything. Because to begin with it's fine. Yes your body's going to be sore. But then you get to the stage where actually, you're tired basically. You're knackered. So when you wake up at 4:30 every morning and start at five, you just think, 'I'm just going to stay in bed today.' Your crew literally have to get you up and get you out. There'll be days when everything is so painful, you just don't want to do anything at all. But you have to move forward. It's really, really hard work. But once you get over the halfway point and you're heading towards the finish, it gets a little easier. You know, you've got a week to go or whatever. You start picking up momentum again. But that's a long way off.

When we did the Marathon des Sables in 2001, halfway through, I was very, very ill. There were three of us running it together and I was really struggling. The two other girls were in front of me and I literally had tears coming down my face just thinking, 'I can't do this.' And I genuinely thought that would be the end and I'd have to pull out and I'd go home, having failed. And one of my team-mates, Max, came up to me, and she just looked to me and said, 'Mimi, think of all those people at home who think you're going to fail'. And then she just walked off. And yes it's harsh, but actually that's when I pulled myself together. And every time I have a bad patch I just think of all those people who really think I'm going to fail and it keeps me going.

Many people I've met at endurance events, especially women in their forties and fifties, have told me how Mimi is an inspiration to them. She's an inspiration to me too, to be honest. And being an inspiration – that must be rather nice.

Yeah, I love it. I love the fact that I get lovely messages from ladies in their sixties, which is not far off for me now. Just saying, I want to go and do Comrades*, I want to try these incredible races. I just think that is fantastic.

---

* The Comrades Marathon, the world's oldest and largest ultra, runs annually between the cities of Durban and Pietermaritzburg in South Africa. It's around 55 miles long. The direction of the race changes each year – everybody says the 'up' run from Durban is easier than the 'down' return from Pietermaritzburg. If you miss the 12-hour cut-off, burly security guards physically form a barrier to stop you crossing the finishing line.

We were written off years ago you know, women when they hit their forties were just written off. And now you've got people in their seventies doing it. But I think really it's because I've been doing it for such a long time; I'm just a granny to the ultra-running world as well.

And I absolutely love how popular the sport has become. You look back to 2000, it's 17 years since I've been running and back then the Internet didn't exist. Most people didn't have computers, let alone laptops. There were no smartphones. There was no information out there about races because there weren't that many. And they've just exploded. You know Centurion have put all those races on, the 100-milers and the 50s and there are all these other races too. You're watching lots of people going in and especially the women. Now you've got 40 women from the UK alone every year doing the MdS. When I did it in 2001, there were 12 of us.

And seeing people finish great challenges, ultras, you know, it's my most favourite thing. Every year I give out the medals at the South Downs Way 50-mile race. And it's a real mixture. You've got the first guys who come in and they're knackered but they're smiley and give great big hugs. But as you get further and further down the field, you have some people who come in and they give you a big hug and they just go, 'I'm knackered.' And I say 'But you've just finished your first 50 – what a massive achievement!' I love that. I will stay from the first person right up to the last person who comes through because they're all as important as each other. In some ways the last person is more important than the first to be honest. I've had people bursting into tears. I remember I handed out the medals a few years ago at an ultra. And I waited. There were these two women who were in five minutes before the cut-off. We were cheering them on as they were coming up to the finishing line. One of them was just gasping and I told her that I thought she needed a hug. She looked completely intense and worried about being all sweaty and filthy. But who gives a damn, that stuff really doesn't really matter. It was a massive achievement for her. Just massive.

Speaking of massive achievements, Mimi rates her remarkable double Spartathlon as one of her own proudest moments. Mainly because two years previously she had failed to beat the cut-offs, and didn't complete the single Spartathlon. Most people don't either. Historically, only around a third of competitors reach Sparta, and for first-timers that proportion drops further still.

But back on the mountain, I'm rather enjoying myself. The top has done its job and warmed me up. I'm alone on a dark mountainside, and revelling in the concentration needed to negotiate the descent. If this were the Dragon's Back Race, you'd class this as one of the easier, more runnable slopes and be swooping down it with abandon. But I've already run over 100 miles, the rocks are slippery, and all around it's pitch black but for the small pool of light emanating from my torch. My legs are beginning to feel trashed, but not dangerously so. I'm being a bit cautious.

I double check my maths and confirm to myself that I've built a five-hour buffer. I'm starting to believe that I won't just finish, but might even finish well. The descent doesn't take too long and I canter through the next few aid stations.

And then my race unravels.

13. paris

Orly airport, Paris, March 2017. The aftermath of an attempted terrorist atrocity. A man attacked a soldier, put a gun to his head saying he wanted to 'die by Allah'. The terrorist was shot and killed, and everybody, staff and passengers alike, immediately evacuated from the airport.

The terminal has only just reopened. Outside, the queue for taxis is truly epic. Hundreds and hundreds of people, frustrated, stressed, late, hauling luggage, overflowing the roped-off waiting area to form an unruly line stretching far towards the car parks. And very few cabs. Optimistically it'll be two hours before I reach the front of the queue, and I simply don't have two hours. I've already missed the start of my race but the organisers – with a Gallic distaste for the morning's attempted atrocity – have told me to come and run anyway. They'll wait for me, as long as I arrive within half an hour.

I've spent the past four hours in a plane on the tarmac waiting to be allowed to disembark. I've flown in for the day to run an excellent-sounding 80km race from the outskirts of Paris to the top of the Eiffel Tower. The attempted terrorism was obviously the lead story on all news bulletins, and during the long delay, as a BBC reporter 'on the ground', I've been giving updates to various TV and radio news channels. I even commandeered the plane's only iPhone charger. In Russia, a doctor friend heard me on the World Service and texted to say hi.

On board the plane, the British Airways crew were doing a grand job. The captain told us what little he knew and opened the door to the cockpit in case anyone wanted to 'have a look around, or come up and chat'. Orly airport, we learned, was 'zero rated' by the security services, whatever that means. Even the pilot didn't know. It definitely wasn't a good thing. The crew served cups of tea and bags of nuts.

Next to me, a man stared wistfully at a jumbo jet on the next stand, just 40 feet away. 'That's the plane I need for my connecting flight to New York,' he told me. 'If I don't make it, I'll miss my subsequent connection to Los Angeles and my important meeting.'

I happened to know there were direct flights from London to LA, and unhelpfully told him as much. 'This way,' he says, 'was slightly cheaper.' A decision he now regretted.

I was looking out of windows at heavily armed security personnel and clusters of flashing blue lights. Occasionally a police car screamed past with lights flashing and sirens blaring. Just as it looked like we were going to be stuck for many more hours, at around exactly the time the Paris Eco-Trail race was setting off, the airport reopened. First staff, then passengers were allowed inside. We gave the BA captain and crew a spontaneous and well-deserved round of applause as we disembarked.

Inside the terminal, as you can imagine, it was utter chaos. I called the organisers of the race to plead my case.

'Yes I know I've missed the start,' I attempted in my best French. 'But I've been caught up in the incident at Orly...'

That's as far as I got.

'Wait by your phone!'

Five minutes later she was back on.

'*Normalement*,' she says, 'there's nothing I could do. But these are exceptional circumstances. I'll hold the race open for you. You say on your entry form that you expect to finish in seven to eight hours... *Bon*, you will still arrive at the Tour d'Eiffel before the close. Just be at the start in half an hour. *Bon course!*' A few years ago, in my late teens say, perhaps even my twenties, I'd have barged straight to the front of the taxi queue, made up some excuse, got into a cab, made the start.

But somehow, as I stand and look at the many thousands of stressed, harassed, impatient people waiting for taxis, it simply doesn't seem right. Bad karma. What makes my race any more important than wherever everyone else is heading? I call the race organiser back, tell her there's no chance of making the start, thank her for trying, and trudge disconsolately towards the metro and my cheap hotel near the finish line.

I phoned the hotel yesterday to warn them not to expect me until late at night. The race doesn't just end at the top of the Eiffel Tower – it ends with a *party* at the top of the Eiffel Tower which all finishers are invited to. I intended to run 50 miles, then enjoy myself. The receptionist looks suitably confused when I turn up 14 hours earlier than advertised. My room's not ready. Of course it's not. This is turning into an expensive fiasco of a weekend.

My flight home isn't until early the following morning, there's 6 Nations rugby on the telly, and I'm sorely tempted to find the nearest bar, watch the sport and drown my sorrows.

The devil on one shoulder is practically dragging me towards beer and rugby, but the angel on the other whispers annoyingly in my ear. *You've come here to run. You've sacrificed a day of your life, a day with your family, to go on a long run. You need a long run in your legs for the huge events you've got coming up, the Dragon's Back Race and the Spartathlon. You can still salvage the situation by simply going for a long run anyway.* Like I say, annoying.

I glance wistfully across the road at the assembled happy throng waiting for Scotland vs Italy to kick off with large glasses of beer in their warm hands. My fingers are numb with cold as I lace up my trainers and set off down the street. I don't really know where I'm heading, only that I want to run for 30 miles at least, preferably 40. My legs feel heavy with the stress of the morning. It's going to be a long afternoon.

What got me out here anyway? Randomly setting off through central Paris on a run likely to last six hours. Less than a decade ago, the idea of 'going for a run' was laughable as I sat in the pub drinking lager, eating crisps and contemplating nothing more strenuous than nipping outside for a cigarette.

It was a mundane roll of tummy fat that first prompted me to do something about my fitness (or lack of it). I'd recently become a father, stopped the smoking, but didn't much like the idea of being overweight. As I drove to work and glanced down, I found to my horror a noticeable spare tyre, a little tube of fat wrapped in a yellow golf shirt and flopping over my belt.

So the choice was clear: diet or gym. Stop eating whatever I wanted or start burning more calories. A tough call, both were equally appalling prospects at the time. But greed beat sloth in the battle of the deadly sins – and later that same day I found myself tentatively arranging a personal training session in Television Centre where I worked. Before too long, treadmill (which I hated) became trail as I borrowed some battered tennis shoes and headed for my first-ever outside run. Which I just loved.

Maybe not that first run, come to think of it. That first run began a little too enthusiastically and I was gasping for breath before I'd even reached the end of my street. But soon running became so much more than an easy way to keep the pounds off. Running sorted me out. Still does.

I've realised that if I'm ever in a funk, or stuck on something, I go for a run and when I get back, that's it, mood improved or problem solved. It's also the best way to stop feeling tired, the best way to give myself some much needed va-va-voom after too many early starts. The mental health benefits are enormous. Like many, I've had my lows. And running gives me space. Both space to think, time to myself, and space in a physical sense – it's whilst running that I feel most deeply connected to a place, whether that be magnificent mountain, fabulous forest or slightly smelly city street.

It didn't come easy. Early on, every run was a struggle. I'd be puffing and hurting within minutes, with an atrocious gait and a string of injuries waiting around the corner. But even through all of that, through the muscle pulls, ankle sprains and ligament tears, I knew I'd stumbled on something life-changing and life-affirming. I didn't have to be especially good at it, but this running thing, I concluded, was a shortcut to a better version of me.

Fitness, therapy, improvement, discovery – many birds with one stone. Speaking of stones, weight loss too. I won't pretend I don't love the fact that I can largely eat what I want – even though my tastes have gotten predictably healthier as my daily mileage has increased.

So I fell head over heels in love with running, and simply stuck with the journey wherever it chose to take me. Early on, it was often to the consulting rooms of various physios and specialists, and to a running school to sort out my appalling gait.

Then it took me to my first start line, the 2010 Great North Run, and a glorious celebration of running and humanity. Such compelling stories among the thousands making the 13.1-mile journey from Newcastle to South Shields. And such generosity and warmth among the million or more spectators lining the route. I was blown away. I was hooked.

I soon progressed to a full marathon and as I crossed the finishing line in Barcelona, decided to find out how much faster I could run if I trained properly. Thus began several happy years punctuated by frequent, single-night minibreaks with my cousin, another Vassos, to run 26.2 miles in weird and wonderful places (Ljubljana, Copenhagen, Bergen...). We'd both developed an unseemly obsession with trying to break the magical three-hour barrier, and had lots of fun along the way. Our trademark was the marathon-eve dinner. Accepted wisdom states you should never eat anything new or unusual the night before a big race, just in case it disagrees with you and you have an upset stomach: tough to run 26 miles with a dicky tummy. We revelled in ignoring that (entirely sensible) advice, beginning in Barcelona with curious Catalan concoctions involving giant onions swimming in oil, sausages the size of your arm and two separate snail dishes. All washed down with a pint or two of Spanish lager. We both ran well the following day, and a tradition was born. Wherever we went we'd sample the local cuisine, the more outlandish the better, and a massive pre-marathon meal became part of our ritual. There was something gloriously decadent about those evenings.

Cousin Vassos graduated from 3:07 (Milton Keynes) to 2:58 (Eindhoven) with barely a hiccup, and promptly lost motivation to keep racing. However, for ages I just couldn't persuade my legs to run 26.2 miles any quicker than 3:02:11. Three hours, two minutes and eleven seconds, the figure tattooed onto the front centre of my mind – those 132 excess seconds taunting me during every training run. I was very jealous of cousin Vassos; at that stage I'd have gladly swapped my running mojo for a marathon PB starting with a two.

It was the treadmill, oddly, that both broke and sorted me out. That and the Lake District. I rarely run inside, but for several months forced myself to do a weekly treadmill 'power hour' in a bid to gain some much-needed pep in the legs. It's the fiendish invention of a coaching pal: four minutes at target marathon pace, one minute flat out sprinting. No rest. Repeat × 12. I feel like throwing up just thinking back to it.

The marathon I'd earmarked to finally break three hours was in Kent, 17 laps of an undulating cyclopark. I was confident I'd put in the training miles, including 10 of those appalling 'power hours'. Then three days before race day I returned to the treadmill for a quick 20-minute 5K to keep the legs turning over. Only somehow, I still don't understand how, I managed to talk myself into a 40-minute 10K blast up a 3% incline. I mean, what was I *thinking*?

I blew up in Kent, of course I did. Ran 3:15. Furious with myself, I returned to the treadmill a few weeks later, determined to put things right. I knew it wouldn't count, doing a sub-3 marathon on a treadmill, but it seemed important to me at the time. And it did then make it easier to do it officially, knowing I had the time 'in my legs'. However, it also showed me how utterly trivial this all was.

At around the same time, I ran a half marathon in Keswick. The one that begins with a boat trip over Derwentwater. My first time in the fells. After the first, seemingly endless climb, I remember cresting a peak and suddenly it was as if my eyes had been freshly opened.

You're on top of England, drinking in the beauty and wilderness. Senses are razor sharp. You just feel so alive! And then you start descending, crazy-quickly down the steep, rough slopes, and that sensation is intensified. You need complete focus, utter absorption. On the rare occasions you get it right, you feel like you're completely at one with your surroundings. You lose yourself in the environment, lose your sense of space and time. Energised, involved, and thoroughly enjoying the experience. And indeed the process. It's as close to what they call 'flow' as I think it's possible for us mere mortals to come. And having lost yourself awhile, later you rediscover yourself refreshed.

Watching the elite fell runners go downhill, now that's something else entirely. Not especially graceful, but astonishingly fast. Their mantra, which will surprise nobody who's seen them in action, is 'brakes off, brain off'. I think part of my trouble during the Dragon's Back Race was overthinking.

That was a seminal run for me in Keswick. Because I'd also been flirting heavily with lots of gadgets, spending too much money on unnecessary equipment. And obsessing unhealthily about the sub-3 marathon. But up in those fabulous fells, I finally worked out that running stops being pleasurable – and stops being a release of tension, stops being an escape, an act of discovery and self-discovery – if you're constantly stressing about how fast you're travelling, what you're wearing, what your heart rate is doing.

The fact is, you're running when you could be walking. It's simple and childlike and brilliant. I once interviewed a sports psychologist with a deeply impressive client list. He quoted Leonardo da Vinci at me. 'Simplicity,' he told me. 'Simplicity is the ultimate sophistication.'

Thus began a love affair with trail running that has only deepened and matured with the passing miles. Not that I don't also enjoy pushing myself hard on the road. The Tuesday evening 10km blast with Barnes Runners has become a staple (and not just because we go to the pub after). I love road running; I live for the trail.

So what on earth I'm doing running aimlessly along a Paris pavement is debatable. The hotel is close to the Eiffel Tower. I decide to follow the river out of the city and just see what happens. At least if I stay by the

Seine I can't get lost. As I run, I see tell-tale signs. Red and white striped tape tied to lampposts and trees or so. *Could this possibly be the race route?* I wonder.

The tape leads me along the river, through a park and surprisingly hilly suburbs. I'm soon in no doubt that I'm doing the backwards. There's still loads of tape marking the route, and then, at the top of a long hill in some formal gardens, an aid station.

I could do with a drink of water and a sandwich, and as a fully paid up member of the race I'm entitled to ask for one. However, my race number's back in my bags so I can't prove my credentials. I consider trying to explain what's happened, but think better of it. In their position, *I* wouldn't believe me. Funny how much more you want something when you can't have it. I realise I've not eaten a proper meal all day, having planned on buying breakfast at Orly airport. Three cups of tea and a British Airways bag of peanuts aren't really fuel for a long run.

I continue through thirst, hunger and some formal gardens, which I discover are part of the Domaine National de Saint-Cloud. It's a former nature reserve, now one of the most beautiful parks in the world. There are Medici lion sculptures casually strewn among yew trees trimmed into perfect triangles. From the hilltops, delightful views over the Parisian cityscape.

The race, as I follow it backwards, passes the grand, brushed bronze dome of the Meudon Observatory, meanders through a forest and heads out towards the palace at Versailles. The leading runner passes me going the other way, swiftly followed by the guy in second.

I'm around 10 miles outside Paris as dusk is falling. I'm just beginning to enjoy myself when I remember my head torch (remember that I've forgotten it). I don't fancy getting lost in the dark, and realise I need to get back to some streetlights pronto. Increasing my pace, I make it to Paris before the moon – just. Back past the aid station, remembering anew how hungry and thirsty I am, back through the suburbs and along the south bank of the Seine towards the Eiffel Tower.

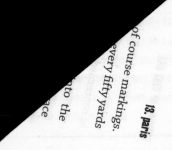

...ed, utterly calorie-deficient, getting by

...thing as far as long-term ultra fitness

...they call it, or running on empty – I'm

...get by on its fat stores – but it's torture.

...still have 10 (or ideally 20) miles of hard

...he hotel where my wallet is, as the lure of

...be overwhelming. Instead I cross the river

and head no... ...le heading out for a Saturday night on the tiles, and through endless plumes of diesel fumes from the permanently gridlocked roads. I'm running, but I'm not going anywhere. I'm simply making up the miles. It's no fun at all.

Occasionally, back home in London, I like to run through the night. I find it kind of soulful. And the next morning, sweaty, exhausted but exhilarated, I arrive at the studio to begin work on the Breakfast Show. When the pavements thin out and there's hardly anybody about, it feels like you've put the city to bed, all tucked up and cosy, whilst you patrol outside. I tend to meander through the parks (which you'd think would be spooky but aren't), along the glorious Thames embankment, and even sometimes dodge the revellers through bustling Soho streets. Once I ran a nocturnal London Marathon – jogging out to Greenwich and recreating the race route as best I could. It was an ace night.

So now, as passers-by give quizzical looks to the guy weaving his way through the crowded Parisian pavements with a pained expression, little do they know that in my head I'm miles away, in a different capital city, running the best road race in the world.

Outside the metal barriers, the crowds are six deep on either side. They're holding up signs, either aimed at someone specific ('Come on Vicky!', 'You can do it Dad!'), or amusing and generic ('All toenails go to heaven', 'Always give 100% – except when giving blood'). Everybody's shouting encouragement. I really do adore London – marathon, city and people.

Not that Paris isn't similarly brilliant. But I'm dizzy with hunger now and the miles are ticking by ever so slowly. Through the grinding discomfort, I keep forcing myself back into the fantasy that I'm running down the happy streets of London in that extraordinary atmosphere. And I keep reminding myself that this is my only chance to get a much-needed long run in; if I don't complete it, I'll have given up a day with the family for nothing.

With four miles to go before I hit the magic 40, I end up back near the hotel. I don't want to get lost and run an inch over the 40 miles I've set as my target, so I end up running around and around the same block. Now people really do look at me like I'm mad. Imagine you're out for dinner on a Saturday night in central Paris and the same bloke just keeps plodding slowly past your window table every two or three minutes.

Those final four miles gave me a tiny glimpse into a truly mind-boggling event – the Self-Transcendence 3100 Mile Race, held annually around the same nondescript block in the New York Borough of Queen's. Almost 6,000 identical laps – around a high school, alongside a freeway and past a small playground. An average of 60-odd miles or 120 laps-a-day, with everyday life going on around you. Every year, several dozen highly committed people choose to do just that – running around the same city block *every single day for two months*. And frequently, they return the following year to do it all over again.

Meanwhile I happily give up running round my Parisian block after about half an hour. Enough self-transcendence for one day. Time for a bath, a beer and bed.

14. frome

'You may be interested to know that you're running today with legend
of triathlon Chrissie Wellington and BBC sports presenter Vassos
Alexander.'

This from the guy with the megaphone at the start of a 50-mile race in
Somerset. The race director, Dave Urwin, has just delivered his briefing
('Course marking may be a bit dodgy – sorry, it's been a hell of a week!')
and is about to set us going along the little-known Mendip Way from
Frome, just south of Bath, to Weston-super-Mare on the coast.

As it happens, the 'legend of triathlon' and the 'sports presenter' had
arranged to run this together, but somehow contrived to enter different
races. So while I stand next to a gate in a quiet Somerset suburb (the
unlikely mouth of the Mendip Way) with a hundred or so other runners,
Chrissie is still at home in Bristol, enjoying a hearty breakfast and
preparing to head for Wells, a picturesque cathedral city where she'll start
the alternative, 30-mile version. We'd somehow got our text messages
muddled. The full-fat Mendip Marauder does pass through Wells, but by
the time I get there Chrissie will be long gone and, awesome as she is,
well on her way to finishing first overall in a ridiculously fast time.

Meanwhile I've been regretting my decision not to upload the GPX
file of the race route onto my Garmin. I'd assumed, wrongly, that the
Mendip Way would be similar to the South Downs Way – well-marked,
well-trodden and basically impossible to get lost on. Especially for
someone fresh from the Dragon's Back Race on the wildest and remotest
terrain in the UK.

Error. The Mendip Way is thoroughly charming, and in parts utterly
beautiful, even captivating – but it's anything but obvious. And I'm
beginning to realise why we were warned in the briefing about the

distinct lack of course marking. I'm in no particular hurry so I'm finding my frequent routing errors amusing, but others aren't so cavalier or forgiving. One American competitor is furious, with frequent East Coast swear words being hurled loudly at the West Country heavens. Very loudly. If you were within a few hundred miles of the Mendip Hills on August 4th 2017, you probably heard her. And swiftly covered your children's ears.

I chat to her for a while as we both converge on the correct path from different, equally penal, wrong turns. It turns out she's a seasoned ultra-runner from Maryland who's finding it hard to come to terms with our occasionally more relaxed approach to the sport in the UK. She tells me how Dean Karnazes himself once presented her with a trophy after she finished third ('podiumed') in a major American ultra and how she's not used to race numbers being handed out on a pavement ('sidewalk') from the boot ('trunk') of a car. She's currently on holiday ('vacationing') in the West Country with her boyfriend, a chain-smoking Italian who'd apparently rather sit on the sofa drinking Chianti and rolling 'special' cigarettes than do anything remotely resembling running. I assume that by special cigarettes, she means joints, and wonder aloud how appalling it would be if she combined their hobbies and attempted to go for a run whilst stoned. But I'm in for a shock. My new friend tells me earnestly how it's her all-time favourite pastime, and how I shouldn't knock it before I try it. I inwardly resolve, equally earnestly, never, ever to try it.

Soon afterwards, the path narrows as it turns uphill through a wood and next time I look round, she's nowhere to be seen. Race director Dave is pleased to inform me when we speak a few days later that by the time she finished, the American was in a much happier mood. But Dave himself is no stranger to dark places.

I live up to many of the ultra-world clichés, coming to the sport from addiction, and I'm also quite 'lonerish' as a person. I was unpopular at school, and sort of retreated into my own shell. I went to alcohol and drugs

149

to find escapism. Obviously that does give you escapism but it also ruins your physical and mental health over time.

I got to a place, when I was about 21, where I had a bit of a meltdown and didn't leave the house for about seven months. But then the thought struck me that if I didn't do something, that would be my life for ever. I'd just be stuck in that house. I just couldn't let that happen.

I don't think I sat there and thought, 'If I do exercise, this is going to get the endorphins flowing, and it might be good for my mental health.' It was more an instinct type thing. Somehow I knew that I had to do something to improve my health. At the time it was just like walking a little bit further from my front door each day. Because when I first started doing that I couldn't walk, literally, down to the end of the street without having a panic attack. So I'd just try and go a little bit further each time. And eventually it got to the point where I could walk a few miles. It took quite a long time after that before it turned into running.

Then when I started going further, I started to feel a bit better. And I realised the exercise was actually helping. I signed up to do the London 10K for Mind, the mental health charity. I'd never run 10K without stopping before, but I managed it. My time was nothing impressive whatsoever. I think it was about 56 minutes. But I really enjoyed it and after that I thought, 'Maybe I can actually run.'

I built up the distance quite quickly. All of these things that just seem crazy in our mind, and seem impossible, once you've actually done them, you think, 'Ah, that wasn't too bad, maybe I could do something else.' To begin with, that London 10K seemed like a ridiculously long way, when I'd never even run half of that before. Once I actually did it I thought, 'Oh, maybe a half marathon could be possible', and when I had done that, 'Maybe I could even do a marathon.' That's how I got into ultras eventually.

When I started running, my mental health improved pretty much immediately. When I first got into it, I was running a lot because I enjoyed it. And it almost became a new addiction in a way, but a healthier one. I think I just had so many endorphins flowing round my system. That did make me feel better overall. I think being able to do something I never thought was possible gave me a lot more confidence and really did boost my overall mental well-being. And just having a focus, something to focus a lot of my time on as well.

Before all of that I'd been spending every day indoors and just feeling anxious and depressed. Obviously running works with both mental and physical health if you push past that initial barrier. Everyone when they start is hobbling round the block and sucking air and not feeling great. But if you just persevere with it, you actually build up more fitness and get better at it. It's going to boost your mental well-being as well. And when you're doing that much exercise, you feel like living a healthier life to go along with it. It all follows. It's a virtuous circle rather than a vicious circle.

When you run really long ultras, you get an amount of thinking time that you just never have in your day-to-day life. Because it's just ridiculously busy nowadays, life. You just don't really get the time to stop and think. Running has always been one of my best ways of doing that. So I think being out for however many hours just in nature and away from all the technology and everything has just taken me back to realising what life is all about.

Realising what I'm capable of as well. A lot of people have said that too. How if you run an ultra, if you complete something that you didn't think was possible, it's amazing what else you think might be achievable. I think that's very true as well. Running has made me a lot more confident within myself. And it's made me believe that things that I thought were ridiculous before, can actually be done.

Dave tells me how he's busy working on several new books, as well as organising half a dozen races every year as head of Albion Running. And I'm thoroughly enjoying this particular event on a summer Saturday afternoon.

I continue on my merry Mendip way, missing turnings here and there, doubling back until I find the right route and generally enjoying the fact that I have nothing else to do today apart from run. Mind you I do find myself wishing my legs felt a little more springy and that my ankle, which I comprehensively trashed in Snowdonia, was a little less hurty. I wonder if I'm doing myself more harm than good by continuing to run on it.

I'm here to get some much-needed miles in my legs ahead of the following month's Spartathlon. But what if I inadvertently rule myself out by aggravating an injury?

This run has been cunningly organised as part of a weekend away with loads of activities planned for tomorrow. My family are meeting me tonight at the seafront finish. I decide the only decent thing to do in the circumstances is to get there. They're being kind enough already; the last thing my wife needs is a phone call begging to be picked up from the middle of nowhere.

Before long, I come to the end of the wooded path and accidentally turn into a farmyard. A man gets off his tractor and approaches. Just as I think he's going to tell me off for trespassing, he cheerfully points me in the right direction. A hundred yards later, I'm lost again. As I retrace my steps I bump into another runner, Nick, who's heading the right way, having been given more extensive directions by the farmer. Nick also has a handheld GPS device, which he describes as his best friend during ultras. For the next few miles, it turns out to be mine too.

How much extra distance I'd have run without Nick and his GPS I have no idea. Definitely half a dozen miles, possibly more. My method of following a combination of my nose and the few-and-far-between bits of red and white tape marking the route would've been ruinous. It had been tough to spot before, but for the next 10 miles or so, even with satellites helping to guide us, we only barely manage to follow the route – frequently going wrong. The Mendip Way is endlessly surprising and rarely predictable. It leads us through high-rise cornfields, between alleyways of stinging nettles, along pathways of trippy tree-roots and down murderously slippy muddy tracks. I lose count of the number of times I almost fall over, and my shins become painful tributes to the flourishing nettles.

I'm absolutely loving it. And extremely grateful for Nick and his GPS. The fact that he's also a tremendously nice bloke is simply a bonus – though not altogether unexpected. As I'm beginning to properly appreciate, people who run – especially people who run ultras – are generally delightful.

Nick won, actually won, his previous race, a 30-miler in nearby Dorset. He's keen for a good finish here too and sets a furious pace. He took several wrong turns at the start and the extra mileage has cost us places. At the very least, he wants to beat his pal James from their running club.

We reach a checkpoint with around 15 miles to go and Nick checks the list of runners who've already been through. To his delight, we're ahead of James. To my delight, I spot our big bronze Land Rover, which means my family are nearby. I hear them before I see them (both my daughters, aged 13 and three, are brilliantly noisy) and their hugs galvanise achy legs.

Now they're here though, I face the conundrum of whether to pull out for the sake of my ailing ankle. The sensible side of my brain says *yes, stop running*. My left knee still hurts most days after I once refused to give in to its protestations during an ironman-distance triathlon. I could do without my right ankle joining the pain party. But the whispering voice in my gut is the one I usually listen to: *you never willingly pull out, your only Did Not Finish was when the Dragon's Back ate you for breakfast. It would begin an unwelcome trend for a second DNF to come in the very next race.*

I carry on.

And what a happy few hours I spend. Running, chatting, jogging, hiking up some surprisingly steep hills. This won't be news to the people of Somerset, but the county is utterly sublime. The spectacular Ebbor and Cheddar Gorges, the punchy climb up to Crook Peak, the incredible views over the Somerset Levels to the circular Cheddar

Reservoir, and England's smallest city, Wells, with its bustling market and magnificent cathedral. Running past the cathedral through that market on a sunny Saturday morning, a full marathon already in the legs, wondering which way to turn through the thronging, bargain-hunting hordes, it's an experience I won't forget in a hurry. An elderly man points the way, before adding, unhelpfully, 'Another runner came past here ages ago – are you sure you're in the same race?!'

All the while, I'm still running with Nick. I'm trying to take things relatively easy to protect my ankle and make sure I'm OK to return to running in a day or two; I can't afford too many recovery days if I have any hope of completing the Spartathlon. Nick meanwhile is intent on overtaking as many people as possible in the hope of a decent finish. And definitely staying in front of the pesky James.

The miles tick by, into single figures remaining now, and I find I'm actually a little disappointed every time my watch buzzes to let me know I'm edging closer to the finish. We try to encourage some of the struggling 30-mile runners as we pass them, and otherwise simply take time to enjoy the journey. After all this is what we do for fun.

Five miles to go, we've been running together for five hours or more now, and I suggest we finish together too. There's the merest second or two of silence. We're both thinking the same thing – shall we just race instead...?

In my mind, I'm thinking that I'm still feeling fresh (fresh being a relative term of course, having just run almost 50 miles) and I'm liking the idea of a challenge. Much as I don't think of myself as competitive, the consensus among friends and family is that I am. I reckon Nick is relishing the idea of a sprint finish: he's just won his last ultra and likes the idea of putting that bloke off the radio in his place. The silence grows.

But then the same thought seems to pierce the bubble as it hits us both simultaneously. It would be churlish to race each other on a day like this. What do we really have to gain, even by winning? We agree to complete together. And for me, however competitive my wife Caroline claims I am, it's the perfect way to finish a long day's running – crossing the line with a new friend.

It seems strange to be thinking of 'tomorrow's easy recovery run' in the middle of an ultra-marathon when you're pushing for a place in the top five, but that's exactly what we're doing, trying to protect against the demon DOMS (Delayed Onset Muscle Soreness). Keeping up a respectable pace whilst not grinding ourselves into the ground for the sake of a few minutes off the finishing time.

It reminds me of the London Marathon a few months beforehand. That day, running under a large arch of red balloons, a surprising thought occurred. Surprising, but quite wonderful. The balloons signalled 21 miles completed, and whilst all around me were grinding their teeth for the final desperate push, what went through my mind was: 'Oh, what a shame, just five more miles to go.'

My wife and kids saw me on the Embankment and confirmed the diagnosis. I was apparently the happy idiot grinning away in a sea of misery. I'd made an unusually sensible decision 14 miles earlier when I realised a PB was beyond me. I'd resolved to forget the watch, slow down a little – and basically, enjoy the experience.

And what an experience! This was my third London, but the first time I properly appreciated the best marathon supporters in the world. So loud, positive, energetic, generous. Nobody forces them to give up their Sunday morning to cheer on a load of Lycra-clad lunatics, to hand out sweets and shout encouragement. But they do it in their millions, and they do it superbly. Restores your faith in human nature. I smiled constantly and dabbed whenever I heard my name. (My 13-year-old daughter was mortified when she saw me dab. Dad dancing is bad enough, dad dabbing beyond appalling.)

Now I can't honestly recommend dabbing, especially if you have a teenage daughter. But dragging yourself out of your watch and into your surroundings? Best thing ever.

Which is why, back in Somerset, I'm a touch sad when we crest a hill and see Uphill Harbour resplendent in the sunshine below. The finish, we know, is just the other side on the sandy beach of Weston Bay. Not too sad, mind. Much as I'm enjoying myself, taking in the views, being in the moment, it will also be nice to stop running and give the ankle a break – it's been hurting more and more every time I put weight on it.

My favourite thing in the whole world is emerging through customs at Heathrow airport after a long trip and seeing my children run to greet me. My second favourite thing is seeing my children run to greet me as I approach the end of a long race. Under glorious, orange skies on the sands of Weston-super-Mare, I'm treated to my second favourite thing in the world.

Mary, aged three, demands immediate attention. She wants to be lifted into my arms, and is. Emily, 13, and Matthew, 11, are both old enough to know how disgusting their dad will be when he's just run continuously for almost nine hours. The last thing they want is a yucky hug. But they're also nice enough not to care – and pile in for a big, tight, sweaty one regardless.

Nick has kids of similar ages, and patiently waits whilst mine are appropriately cuddled, kissed and carried. All five of us then cross the finishing line together only, horror of horrors, to see Nick's friend James grinning away at him with a medal round his neck. We're joint seventh. He was five minutes in front of us in fourth. There wasn't any tape to mark the final five miles and it seems we may have been overtaken as we unknowingly went the long way round.

The kids are gasping for the fish and chip dinner we promised them this morning, so I don't have time to hang around for a debrief. However, after going slowly to protect my ankle I do feel largely responsible for the failure to finish in front of James. I apologise profusely via text. Nick's very good about it, principally because, in his words, 'he challenged me to a few games of pool in the pub after – and all even, honour satisfied!'

And the fish and chips, by the way, were the business.

15. tegea

I first realise there may be a major problem as I approach the delightful village of Tegea. It's still night time in Greece, the darkest part just before the dawn, which means there's no chance to enjoy the remains of the ancient temple to the goddess Athena. No chance to enjoy very much at all to be honest. My race has started falling apart.

This is one of the few aid stations offering hot food, which I'd been looking forward to. Under normal circumstances some slightly congealed spaghetti would go down a treat after 23 hours' solid running. But I have a grim expression and leaden legs.

Crews are here too. This is an endurance challenge for them as well and they're coping admirably against the escalating fatigue. Russ, who lent me his T-shirt at dusk, is still going strong at dawn. Still smiling. Still full of beans. Amazing really.

'What's up, pal?' He's noticed my grimace.

'My legs are seizing up. Struggling to run at all.'

'Have you taken on board enough salt?'

'I think so, yes.'

I honestly haven't got a clue about the salt. I read an article just before flying to Athens which said salt deficiency is a prime cause of ultra races going awry, so I bought a big pack of one-a-day salt tablets and tipped the lot into my race belt. I know I've eaten plenty, but can't remember when the last one was. I swallow two more, just in case.

Russ then tells me he knows how to reinvigorate my legs. Despite the fact that I'm sweaty, dirty, disgusting, he stands behind me and wraps his arms around my chest.

'Right then,' he says. 'Ten squats please. I'll help you up and down.'

When you've been awake all night, it can't be a pleasant experience to take the weight of a grimy, smelly stranger as he attempts 10 sore squats. Can't be especially pleasant any time, come to think of it. But Russ is a diamond. Another in this sport. Yet another.

He laughs and jokes throughout, and when I eventually leave the checkpoint, my mood has lightened. The sky is about to do the same. If only my legs would follow suit.

Running is no longer an option. It's not a pain thing; I can take pain. It's an impossibility thing. I simply am not able to run any more. I'll ready myself, fortify mind and body, attempt a squat to get the hamstrings going... then stagger forwards a couple of paces before grinding back into a walk. What's going on? This has never happened before.

I keep trying, but a familiar, pathetic pattern emerges. Harden resolve, then – steady, squat, stagger, slow, stop. Repeat. It's like somebody's filled me with concrete from the waist down. And still more than a marathon left to go.

I can't possibly fail from here can I? Even though the cut-offs have eased and the organisers are giving us more time to get from checkpoint to checkpoint, I find myself losing more and more of my precious buffer every time I reach an aid station. I'm wading through time with concrete legs, and I can't keep up.

I stop to stretch at the side of the road. I try everything: hamstrings, quads, groin, calves, even glutes. As I'm finishing off, hanging off a street sign for balance, a kindly German runner stops in front of me.

'What you need is my emergency magnesium,' he says, rummaging in his belt. His hand emerges clutching a tiny bottle with a medical label. He passes it to me with a knowing smile.

'Try this,' he insists. 'It will help.'

'Thanks, but what if you end up needing it?'

'Don't worry about that. Also it is less weight for me to carry!'

And with that he's off. I down the contents of the vial, and await the promised improvement. It doesn't come.

According to numerous race reports I've read, previous Spartathletes writing up their experiences online, the morning brings fresh impetus. It's having the opposite effect on me. All hope seems to seep out of me.

I can feel a heavy mood closing in, enveloping from every direction. My senses are dulled. Everything becomes blurred.

I try desperately to work out if I can walk in from here and still manage to reach the statue inside the mandatory 36 hours. The maths proves too tricky for my addled, sleep-deprived brain. I suspect I cannot. The temptation to stop becomes overwhelming.

I know the mantras, know all the tricks of breaking down a race into manageable chunks. Don't focus on the daunting distance remaining, in this case the many, miserable miles. Concentrate instead on the small stuff: the next aid station, the next road corner, the next tree, the next footstep if you have to. I even practise it during 5K parkruns when the thought of another eyeballs-out kilometre seems outrageous. I know it, I try it now – but it simply doesn't work.

The darkness inside is beginning to overwhelm me. It's new, this, and terrifying. It's begging me to stop, insisting that I stop.

Time is ticking by agonisingly slowly. Even my watch is mocking me. I want to hurl it to the side of the road, but it's got me trapped in its hypnotic movement. I'm checking it every few seconds. I can feel tears of pure self-pity prickling in the corners of my eyes. It's all gone wrong, and all so quickly. Ironic, how the decline can happen so fast, and yet now how every unhappy minute is lasting a lifetime.

A good friend of mine was once involved in a horrible car crash. Fortunately he walked away. But from the moment he first realised there was trouble, all the way through to the upside down aftermath, the entire episode wouldn't have lasted more than five seconds. And yet he told me he could write a book about each of those seconds. He could open them up, stretch them, peruse them. Every one had a story to tell.

It's how I feel now. But there are just so many seconds. So very many. I watch them from above, and steel myself to dive into every one. I'm now fantasising about stopping. Everything's gone gruesome.

Suddenly I know with every fibre of my being that I will not reach Sparta. I will not kiss the statue. What on earth possessed me to think that I could? This race, getting to the finish, it isn't going to happen for me. It can't happen any more. Won't happen. I know I'm going to fail and disappointment – pure, childlike misery – wells up inside me.

Only, I'm no quitter. I'm not giving up without a fight. Like all ultra-runners, I have a capacity to endure, it goes with the miles. One final effort to flip the script. I've had an old Winston Churchill quote going round in my head since somebody told it to me yesterday. 'In future,' the great man growled during the Second World War, 'we won't say that Greeks fight like heroes, but that heroes fight like Greeks.' I'm under the Greek flag today, representing the motherland. *Fight on*, I tell myself. *At least until the next aid station.*

It's enough, just, to keep me putting one foot in front of the other. All the way I consider only the shameful bliss I'll feel when I hand in my race number. Eventually, I reach the checkpoint. By sheer chance, it's one of two or three aid stations staffed by physios offering massages to needy competitors. Could this be the thing that breathes some desperately needed life into my legs? I'm not asking for much life – just a tiny bit please, just the faintest pulse.

I lie down on the table and two kind souls start pummelling my thighs. I close my eyes, but hastily reopen them; I was a nanosecond from falling asleep. The massage feels epic. A minute goes by, two minutes, three... I know I should think about getting up and getting on with it, but the sensation of lying down is utter bliss. I never want the massage to end. More than that, I never want to get up again. The thought of re-entering the race is truly appalling.

The decision is taken from me. The massage ends and I force myself to stand up. I know immediately that the whole thing has been a mistake. Previously, walking took a Herculean effort. Now standing up is ambitious.

The dark mood descends with interest. Here it comes then, the sorry end.

'Just hand in your race number,' says a voice in my head. And then, louder: 'You know it's going to happen, whether it's here or three miles down the road at the next checkpoint. And for what? Does it make any difference where you grind to a stop? Because you sure as hell aren't making it as far as Sparta.'

I look at the volunteers, about to cave in to the urge to remove the safety pins attaching my race number to my shorts. I remember the Churchill quote, but swiftly dismiss it. He was talking about a proper war, proper battles. To compare that to this, a trivial race, is insulting. Anyway, heroes might fight like Greeks and vice versa, but I was born in London.

And actually, it's a very British trait that keeps me moving forwards. I realise it would be rude to the physios to withdraw after their efforts to help me. Not to mention a little awkward. So I thank them – 'efharisto' – and hobble onward.

The Greek word reverberates around my head. *Efharisto*. A quiet, humble corner of my mind clasps that gratitude, embraces it, holds on to it. A tiny glimmer of positive emotion to combat the tidal wave of negativity that had been drowning me. But it's enough.

A modicum of resolve returns. Perhaps I won't make it to Sparta, perhaps these wasted legs of mine aren't able to propel me the remaining miles fast enough. But I suddenly know for damn sure, they're going to try.

Ever since I started running ultras, I've harboured a small, secret suspicion. That people pull out of endurance races prematurely and/or petulantly. I've always thought I'd never be guilty of that. But suddenly I get it. The mind is all that matters. When that goes, when the pernicious questions start, it's a very short step to surrender. Traces of the darkness still linger, a nasty aftertaste. I'm embarrassed by my earlier thoughts of quitting.

I now know with absolute cast-iron certainty that I'm all in. I'll doubtless fail, but I won't give up – however much it hurts my body and however black my mood. It's simultaneously liberating and terrifying. I plod onwards, one painful step at a time.

The thought occurs that the winner will have reached the statue by now, and the church bells of Sparta will have pealed in pre-dawn acclamation. I find myself wondering if any of the British team have made it yet. I later discover that Nathan Flear, a likeable Welshman I'd met at registration, was the first British runner to finish.

The previous day as we queued together, he'd had a confident smile on his face and the relaxed demeanour of the accomplished athlete. Something about the way he held himself, he just gave off that air of quiet assurance you often notice in elite sportspeople. Even his tread seemed light. I wasn't in the least surprised when he told me that he'd auto-qualified for the Spartathlon (hadn't needed to go through the lottery for a place as he was more than 20% better than the stringent criteria needed to enter). Also I wasn't surprised when I found out later how fast he'd reached Sparta, in just 27 hours. What did surprise me however, shocked me even, was the fact that two years ago Nathan was severely overweight and had never run a step. Only two years? By any standards, the transformation is astonishing.

Yeah, I was 16-and-a-half stone, smoking 40 a day, drinking a lot. I hadn't done any exercise for 15 years. Nothing. And even at school, I played a bit of football and a bit of rugby, but nothing really. I lived abroad in Spain for nine years, and my life was sedentary, just doing all the wrong things, and getting into bad habits. I just put all this weight on, got really unfit and unhealthy. Then we moved, had children, lived in Bulgaria for a couple of years. We returned here to the UK four years ago, and I started brewing my own beer. I'd always wanted to brew beer.

So I'm brewing beer, I'm having two or three pints every night, and the weight just piled on. And there were all these other comfort foods as well. I'm vegetarian now, but at the time I wasn't, and I was eating pork pies and just crap. We went to Bulgaria that Christmas and people would say to me, 'Oh, your wife is feeding you! You're big!' That was when I realised.

On January 1st, right at the start of 2015, I thought: 'That's it, I'm going to run'. I just decided to lose this weight by running. I did a mile down hill, and walked back up. I kept at it and every day, increased. I threw myself into this running in quite a big way. I'm a marketing consultant, and it affected work. But I was reading all these magazines and books about running and about three months after I started, I read about the Spartathlon. I thought, 'Wow, this sounds amazing.' But then I read you have to qualify to get in. I looked again on someone's blog, and they said it's getting so popular that you've got to get the auto-qualifier because the ballots are so full. And I decided literally three months after I started running, right, my first goal is to run for Wales, and the second goal is to get into this Spartathlon.

When I said it, I don't think anyone really took it seriously. But I believed. Six months after I started, before I'd even run a marathon, I entered a 50K. The Chiltern Challenge. At the time I was probably about 13 stone and it was just brutal. It took me about six hours – even though looking back it's quite a nice course to put a fast time on. But I really enjoyed it. I was eating the cake and sandwiches at the aid stations, and thinking, 'This is great!' When I finished, I realised I had a lot of work to do to get the Spartathlon time. But then I just stuck at it. I represented Wales in the 100K. And finally, at the Robin Hood 100-miler, I thought, 'Right, I'm going to try and get 15 hours to get into the Spartathlon.' And basically, that's what I did.

As we're chatting – and he's making it all sound so easy – I find myself wondering whether the goals I've been setting myself are too modest. Then I remember my despair after 130 miles of the Spartathlon. And I suspect Nathan's race went pretty much perfectly to plan.

Well, no. You know what? It's difficult, because I wanted to go under 24 hours. But that went on the mountain. Everything was going great, my splits, I wanted to finish the first marathon in about 3 hours 15. And then I wanted to reach 100K in 8-and-a-half hours, which I did, bang on. And 100 miles, I was thinking, get to that mountain base between 15 and 16 hours, and I got there in 15:20. So up until that point I was feeling great. But then the mountain.

My head torch went so I had no light and I had to borrow one off somebody. The rain came so I was wet, freezing cold. I slowed right down going up. The ascent just went on and on and on…. And then coming down the other side, I was just terrified of falling. I kept thinking that I didn't

163

want to fall and ruin my race. I decided not to take any risks, so I cranked down and I was getting overtaken by loads of people. That implanted the negative seed I guess. I was starting to slow and it was wet and cold.

I got to the bottom and it was just tough all the way in. The last half marathon, I couldn't run for longer than a mile. Then it was half a mile, then a quarter. I would run for a few hundred yards and stop to squat. Then I'd walk for a minute and then I'd run again for maybe a quarter of a mile and squat again. And this was just never ending. Stopping, walking, squatting. I got to that checkpoint, checkpoint 65, the one with a half marathon to go, and that was where Tori, my partner and my support crew, was waiting for me for the final time. I gave her my jacket and water bottle and I put my British Spartathlon top back on because I had taken it off through the night. And I thought: 'Just a small uphill left then I'm just going to go for it all the way downhill to Sparta, I'm going to run this fast now, and really push on.' But no, it didn't happen. That last half marathon took me three hours, and lots of people overtook me. But I soon stopped worrying about time and position.

I told myself not to care about the clock, and just to finish. And when you get to that statue, and even afterwards, you think well, did it really go wrong? Not really. The only way it could've gone wrong for me is had I not finished. Just finishing the Spartathlon is the thing. It's just amazing.

And when you think about it, it's just a road race. Parts of it are quite ugly, and it goes on for 153 miles, and if you take the people out of it, then it's not that much of a race. But the organisation, the other runners, the children off school asking for autographs in the night, the villages coming out, the whole experience when you finish… it's the people that make the Spartathlon so special.

Back on the long, lonely road to the statue and I'm existing moment to moment. I fear that the final moment – the one when I can no longer take a forwards step – is just around the next corner. I'll battle on until it arrives.

Suddenly, a friendly pat on the shoulder and a ridiculously welcome greeting wrapped in an Aussie accent.

'Hello mate!'

'Mick! You're still in!'

It turns out my roommate from Athens has been as close to quitting as I was. Last time I saw him some 65 miles ago, his stomach problems were preventing him eating or drinking anything. He couldn't run at all, so had resorted to walking as fast as his stomach would let him. Imagine this – you're 70 miles into a race with 83 remaining. Your insides are convulsing. Every time you try to run, you have to squat behind a bush to relieve yourself. Every time you try to replace the lost nutrients, you're back behind another bush. It's chronic food poisoning at the worst possible time. What do you do?

Eventually you bow to the inevitable, right? After a dozen or more trips behind a bush, you realise it's not to be. Extremely unfortunate and all that, but that's your race finished.

Not Mick. Literally and metaphorically, Mick has gutsed it out. When running, eating and drinking were all impossible, he chose the only option remaining (apart from quitting) – he walked onwards in the hope that his stomach situation might improve. Which it did not, for six hours. That's six hours. All night basically, Mick simply carried on as best he could, unable to eat, drink or run. Hoping, just hoping. Eventually he sipped some water and it stayed down. Then a gel. Finally he experimented with running again and gradually upped the pace.

And it's all come good. He may not finish in the sort of time he was hoping for, but the fact he's going to finish at all is testament to his fighting spirit.

He asks why I'm going so slowly. I explain about my loss of leg power. Mick's an experienced ultra-runner and quickly goes through a checklist of what might be wrong:

'Have you taken on board enough salt?'

'Yep.'

'Have you tried doing squats?'

'Yep.'

'How about forcing yourself into a run to see if you can jog some life back into your legs?'

'Yep.'

'Massage?'

'Yep.'

'Stretching?'

'Yep.'

'Magnesium?'

'Yep.'

A pause. I'm hoping he may be about to come up with a miracle cure. 'In which case you're doomed, mate!'

Ah.

Mick's quick to add that he means 'doomed' in a good way. Sort of. He assures me that I can definitely still finish, but that reaching Sparta, if I manage it, is really going to hurt. I could have told him that.

But finding out that Mick's still in the race further reinforces my positive mood. We're heading up a modest hill and several Spartathletes overtake us. This has become such a common occurrence for me, I think nothing of it. But I sense Mick's itching to retake those places. I send him on his way, asking him to save a seat in the closest bar to the statue. I harden my resolve to get there. The beers will be on me.

16. ryde

'Would you mind if I take the kids to my sister's house for the weekend? David's away, so Katie and I thought we could have a mums' day with all the cousins and then a proper catch-up when they're in bed.'

This from my wife Caroline, over a glass of wine one Thursday evening at home.

'Just to be clear. You're asking if I mind you leaving me at home with nothing to do, no kids to look after and no errands to run – for an entire weekend?'

This is me, scarcely believing my luck.

'Not a whole weekend, no. We'll be back on Sunday morning.'

'So all of Saturday then?'

'Yes, all of Saturday.'

'Erm. No I don't mind at all. You carry on.'

I won't pretend I wasn't tempted by the pub and the sofa. Sorely tempted. But I'd had a longstanding urge to run around the Isle of Wight – actually any island, but the Isle of Wight is the most convenient and manageable – and this seemed like the perfect opportunity.

So Saturday morning dawns with Caroline and the kids heading for Sussex in the car, and me on the 6:15 ferry from Portsmouth to Ryde. (Does anyone ever get on that ferry, and *not* sing, 'I've got a ticket to Ryde' over and over in their heads?) My travel companions are some earnest cyclists already on the gels. I suspect they have a similar agenda, only on wheels.

There's something wonderful about running around an island. I've done it once before, on holiday in Thailand, one of the most glorious mornings I've ever spent: up at dawn to the sound of the waves and out into an orange sunrise, past beaches, palm trees and rice fields, through a busy market and a rainstorm, making friends with the English teacher at the tiny local school, and being invited back with the family the following day when all the island children performed a song just for us while our Emily and Matthew, then aged seven and five, reciprocated by reciting a poem. All in view of the clear blue waters of the Gulf of Thailand. The Isle of Wight has a lot to live up to.

According to my research online, the coastal path is 67 miles long, some 50 miles longer than my Thai escapade. Almost all of it hugs the coastline. I'm reckoning on a run of about 10 hours, which is far longer than anything I've attempted outside of an official ultra-race. But I like the poetry of circumnavigating an island on foot, and there's something rather fine and fabulous about setting off on a lone running adventure. No need to register, pin on a number or make small talk at the start. No nervous energy, no jostling for position, no timing chips. Just the simplicity of running for the sake of it. A chance to reflect.

I set off clockwise from Ryde. I've not brought any maps nor loaded a GPX file onto my watch. According to the Internet, the path is well signposted. Just look for the white gulls against blue backgrounds.

It's a grey sort of day, hardly the ideal conditions to appreciate the island's treasures. The first one I reach is called Appleby Tower. There's nobody about as I run past. It looks exactly like a colossal rook from a giant's chess set. Soon I'm alongside some expensive-looking beach huts and idly wonder what's the most money ever paid for a British beach hut. I gleefully realise that I can simply stop running and look it up. This clearly couldn't happen in a race. (Since you ask, it's a whopping £275,000 for a beach hut in Mudeford Spit in Dorset with no electricity, running water or toilet. For the same price you could buy two three-bedroom cottages with an acre of land in the comely village of Maerdy, South Wales.)

Past the large seafront houses of Seaview, where we once spent a holiday when Mary was learning to walk and suddenly took off on grass. The memory of her wildly whirling feet as I lowered her onto a lawn for the first time makes me bark out loud in delight. I'm loving this.

The signposts start sending me inland but I'm not ready to leave the sea so I ignore them. I'm running towards a thin channel of water which I'm convinced I'll find a way across: a bridge, or even just splashing through – it looks barely ankle-deep. Wrong on all counts as it turns out. Suitably chastened, I retrace my steps and resolve to simply follow the white gulls. This run is plenty long enough without extending it needlessly.

The next thing I wonder (and look up) is the distance around mainland Great Britain. It's 5,000 miles. Imagine running all the way round that. Starting in the bottom right-hand corner and heading west along the south coast to the cliffs of Cornwall, then around Wales, up the north-west of England, over Scotland, which is a lot bigger than you think, down the east coast, round East Anglia and back to Kent. Now imagine doing it on your own in your early twenties with all your belongings on your back.

Meet Elise Downing. When she was 23, she quit her job and did exactly that. You won't be surprised to learn that when you talk to her, she's sparkly and bubbly.

I was sitting at work one day, looking at a map, and I wondered, 'Oh, I wonder if anyone's run around the coast before.' At that point, as far as I could tell, nobody had. Then I told a few people I might do it and suddenly, it was this thing that was happening! I don't think it really sank in until I was on the start line and actually had to do it.

I started in Greenwich by the Maritime Museum. About 20 people came to see me off, which was really nice. My mum and dad both came. The first day, running 17 miles to Dartford, was not scenic at all. When I was planning to do this trip, I thought it'd be all lovely and sunshine. But it was foggy, and we were just running along the horrible bit of the Thames in the fog to Dartford. But it was quite fun. It was just like a day out with friends.

I do remember thinking, 'Gosh, this is quite hard. How am I going to run any further than this?' My parents ran with me again the next day, and then we got to Gravesend, and that was when they headed home, and I realised that I was on my own. Then I had a bit of a wobble. I think the main reason I didn't give up there and then was because I was embarrassed as I'd told everybody what I'm going to do. So I should probably hold on at least more than one day.

And then, yeah, it was weird. I don't think it ever really became routine because it changed so much, like the distances and the terrain and the places were all so varied and the weather, it never really became a routine. It always changed. I think it probably took about two weeks for me to say, 'Ah, this is what I'm doing now.'

I took a tent with me, and I thought I'd be camping all of the time. But I camped less than a third of the time in the end because just so many nice people put me up. I'd generally run on my own in the day, and then towards the evening, I'd meet up with whoever had really kindly let me stay. I'd generally spend the evening with them, so the evenings were super varied because I'd be doing whatever my nice hosts decided we were going to do.

I always had great intentions of setting off at like seven in the morning, and it invariably never happened, and I'd still be dithering around about 10 or 11, and I would eventually start running. And yeah, I was kind of on repeat. Social media had a massive part in it and quite a few different hostels and hotels gave me a room in the winter when it was quiet.

For ages, I was really scared about running around Scotland. I don't know why. I just thought Scotland was going to be absolutely terrifying. It was actually nowhere near as remote as I thought. But I told myself, if I got to the Scottish border, then I was allowed, if I wanted, to cycle around Scotland and make it a duathlon. I don't know if I ever would have done that, but just having that in my mind as a get-out-of-jail card really helped motivate me. When I got there and crossed the border, I just didn't really think about it again. I just carried on running.

Finishing was a bit weird because I'd planned the day I was going to finish but I'd put in a few buffer days because I was scared I wouldn't make it in time. As it happens I did make it in time, so I had a day off the day before, which felt ridiculous. I thought I should get to the finish line all broken and tired, and I actually felt fine.

It was a really sunny day, and some friends and family were there, and we had a picnic. It was lovely. Then I went out for a curry and the next day we went to the Notting Hill Carnival. It was surprising how quickly normal life resumed.

When I started this, I really wasn't a very good runner, didn't have much experience and hadn't done any big ultra-races or anything. But I realised that it really didn't matter. It's okay to have a bit of a stupid idea. The amazing thing is, it wouldn't have mattered even if I hadn't been able to finish.

Now I give talks about the fact that you don't have to be great at something to enjoy doing it. And you don't really need to have a clue about what you're doing because I definitely didn't. And I'm petrified of all farm animals, which was problematic, I found, because there are cows everywhere.

I'm pleased to report I've encountered no farm animals so far on the Isle of Wight. I'm secretly scared of cows too. Why do they all gather near the gate or stile you need to get to? And what's the deal with cows with horns? I wish I'd never been told this (and I've looked it up, it's true) but five people are killed by cows in the UK every year. That's five people every year *killed by cows*? How can I approach any field with a cow in it and *not* think about that? Runners from London with no real clue about cow etiquette must be quite high on the danger list. Today I sincerely hope the only cows I come across is Cowes, the town on the north coast of the island.

Right now I'm on the eastern tip. I've reached some cliffs high above a sandy bay. I see a small cafe and decide to stop for breakfast. I start chatting to a couple on holiday; they're friendly, inquisitive, and pronounce me deeply weird for wanting to spend my day off running around an island.

I get this a lot. *Running such long distances, you must be mad!* But am I really? There are clearly other options available to me today, sofa and pub being high on the list. But what's so good about a day that I'll barely remember tomorrow, let alone years later? And fitness-wise, is it more sane to spend your time in the gym, running on a treadmill, going nowhere, seeing nothing? There's a quote I like from Abraham Lincoln. 'In the end it's not the years in your life that count, it's the life in your years.'

The Downs on the Isle of Wight are among my favourite places to run in the world. This is what I've really been looking forward to. I once ran past an elderly man here, he was walking his dog near the Tennyson Monument and remarked how happy and effortless I looked as I ran, and how I reminded him of his younger self. I remember thinking how running seemed to be connecting me both with my surroundings – the pristine cliffs on one side and the rolling hills falling away sharply towards the sea on the other – and with the past. Not much will have changed here in hundreds of years, I thought then, and ponder anew today. Thirty years ago it would have been the elderly dog walker running on these same grassy hills, tripping over the same rocks. And earlier still, his parents and grandparents. What would they have been thinking as they surveyed the magnificent Needles, the huge white rocks jutting out of the sea at the western edge of the island? What were their worries and concerns? Did they too run for the simple joy of it? Did they ever decide to run around the island?

And if the answer to that last question is 'yes', then were they also feeling as knackered as I am now? Were they tempted, as I am, to just jack it in and take a taxi (horse and cart in those days) back to the boat? I've now run the entire south coast, through the touristy town of Shanklin, past two bays within a mile of each other both named 'Horseshoe Bay', along the sea wall into the town of Ventnor and through a lonely stretch of gloriously unspoiled coastline around to the village of Brook (where we also once rented a holiday cottage).

Perhaps it's the thought of a cosy cottage that's giving rise to these second thoughts. It's afternoon now, I'm tired, struggling for motivation and both legs feel leaden. Also, I'm hungry. Properly famished; I haven't eaten anything since breakfast. I resolve to run as far as the next available food, then re-evaluate. However, on the way I realise – that there's no way I'm going to take a taxi and return home disappointed simply because I'm tired. I'm going to finish what I started.

As soon as I stop fantasising about aborting the whole adventure and re-commit, a clumsy sort of spring returns to my gait. And as soon as I find something to eat a smile returns to my lips. I'm so hungry I devour most of the main courses in a cafe, to general astonishment.

Blood sugar levels suitably restored, I thoroughly enjoy running along the north coast of the island, even through aching legs. My quads aren't shredded, but they're not far off. On an inland road I join a couple out for a Saturday evening jog. They don't seem remotely surprised by what I'm up to and tell me it's not uncommon for people to try running (or walking) around the island. Most do stay the night before and after.

I run the final few miles to Ryde fighting a slight trepidation that I've failed to check when the last ferry returns to the mainland. I needn't worry. I make it with hours to spare and even allow myself a self-satisfied grin. The number of islands I've run around is now up to two.

The following day, Sunday, I wake early. It's four hours before Caroline and the kids are due home. Even I'm a little taken aback by my choice of activity: I decide to go for another run. But the thing is, I've just been chatting to the brilliant Ben Smith, who ran 401 marathons in 401 days, raising over a quarter of a million pounds for anti-bullying charities in the process. And doubtless propelled by the endorphins from yesterday's adventure, I'm curious to find out what it's like to run long on consecutive days. *When am I next going to get the chance?*, I reason. That, and the fact that it's meant to be really good if you're, say, planning to attempt the Spartathlon.

I first met Ben on the start line of a marathon, and then again the following morning when he came in to Radio 2 for an interview. If I thought my sub-3 hour time was an accomplishment, I needed to look no further to reclaim some humility. Ben had also run well, his 250th marathon in as many days, with number 251 to come later that morning. Followed by another 150, day after day after day, culminating in a joyous mass celebration in his home town of Bristol.

It was 5th October 2016, Millennium Square in Bristol, I remember rocking up in the morning to the final day, realising that literally 26.2 miles later I would have completed what I'd set out to complete. We'd already achieved three of our four objectives. We'd inspired thousands of people, we'd challenged them to do new things, and we'd raised awareness of bullying. The only thing that we hadn't done was hit our financial target, £250,000.

That final day, we had over 450 people turn up. It was chaotic, but there was a real buzz. I was in a bit of a daze. All I knew was I needed to run. I remember setting out on the course, which was quite poignant because it was the same tracks I learned to run on. It seemed quite symbolic that I used that as my final marathon. I remember running along the towpath, underneath the Clifton Suspension Bridge with 450 people of all different abilities, all dressed in 401 gear. Everybody was together that day in what we were trying to achieve.

I arrived in Portishead and it was a beautiful, sunny day. We couldn't have asked for any better weather. The world's media was there. We were doing interviews everywhere. It just seemed like there was a complete media hype about what we were about to achieve. When we got to halfway, I remember being told the news that we'd just hit the £250,000 mark. Still to this day, I get quite emotional about it. I remember crying live on Sky News, which was extremely embarrassing. From an idea, from just a tiny small idea, we'd achieved something impossible. We'd achieved something that nobody else had, which actually made the final 13.1 miles quite relaxing and I could just enjoy them.

The last mile of the last marathon, 30 primary school kids ran with us. That really summed up what this project was about: inclusivity. It was about inspiring the future generation to think differently about things. I remember crossing that finishing line and I was surrounded by kids from the primary school, people that had come out and supported us right the way through the project. It was a moment that will stick with me for the rest of my life.

Since then, Ben's won numerous awards including the Helen Rollason Award – for outstanding achievement in the face of adversity – at the BBC Sports Personality of the Year. Also Fundraiser of the Year at the Pride of Britain Awards and the Prime Minister's Points of Light Award for outstanding individual volunteers who make a change in their community. It's been quite a journey.

To be perfectly honest with you, finding running was more of a shock to me than anybody. Four years ago I didn't even run. I got into it, I suppose, by accident. It was a friend of mine that spoke up. He was sick and tired of me moaning and groaning about the fact that I should get fit and healthy, because I'd suffered from what they call a TIA, a Transient Ischaemic Attack (a sort of temporary stroke) about a year before. That made me sit up and realise that my life had to change, but I didn't know how that was going to happen. I was 16-and-a-half stone and a 30-a-day smoker. My confidence and self-esteem were at rock bottom. It doesn't happen overnight. I had to figure out what made me happy.

A friend introduced me to my local running club. I remember turning up on the first day and thinking, 'I don't belong here. How can this fat guy run?' I'd never even liked running. I'd never liked sports. This just was not me. But something in my head just pushed me to do it, I tell you: that first night I ran, well mostly walked, three miles. There was a sense of pride inside myself. It was a warm feeling that I'd achieved something I'd never done before. I really liked that feeling.

Obviously, I wanted more of that, so I kept on going. I kept going every week, every week, and I grew to love running. It was tough to begin with, don't get me wrong. And there were days where I was just like, 'Oh, no, I don't want to do this any more.' But I kept at it, and my confidence grew. My self-esteem grew. I grew as a person. I grew into liking myself again. Especially from a mental health point of view, it seemed to be my opportunity to escape and to rid myself of all the stress that I had in my life. It's a cliché but it was a way to find myself again, find who I really was.

I got to travel the world with it. I made a choice in 2014 to run 18 marathons all around the world. I got to reignite my passion for life, and that's why I run. That's why I do what I do. The two anti-bullying charities that I picked, Stonewall and Kidscape, they were extremely close to my heart. They both supported people that went through the things that I went through. To twin the two things that I loved in life, it just seemed like a no-brainer.

So the next question to Ben – which is especially pertinent to me as I embark on a four-hour run the morning after running 67 miles around the Isle of Wight – is, 'What's it like doing a long run, day after day?'

What you can do is take every day as it is. Train as you're doing it. I suffered. Progressively over the first couple of weeks, my body had to adapt to what I was asking it to do. You can't train for 401 back-to-back marathons. My left knee doubled in size. I got severe tendonitis in my left shin. I lost the feeling in my left foot. I fractured a big toe. That was all within the first couple of weeks. But after about 50 days my body started to settle down.

I lost a lot of weight. I lost 17 kilos and my body fat plummeted to the degree where I could literally feel my stomach was cold. The visceral fat levels in my body were minimal. I had to teach myself to eat and run at the same time. I wasn't taking on enough calories. I was following a carbohydrate-heavy diet, which didn't work for me, so I switched that to a high fat, high protein diet, which then caused mood swings.

After about 100 days it switched from being physical into more of a mental game. Finding stuff that motivated me every day. I'm not going to lie, food and coffee motivates me, and the occasional Thatcher's cider. Introducing that, and also knowing the fact that I cheer people on took my mind off my pain and really helped me move forward.

I think the reason why our project was successful is because people opened their hearts to it. People recognised that we were doing this for genuine reasons. It wasn't about becoming famous or becoming the best at something. We genuinely wanted to try to make a difference.

I have a really good friend now, Susie, who I met during the challenge. She runs for Teignbridge Trotters down in Newton Abbot. I met her on day nine. Now Susie, she won't mind me saying this, was a bit overweight. She had just got into running, and she came out and ran with me on that day and she ran further than she'd ever run before. You could see on her face that it was a struggle, but you could also see that she started to have that feeling that I once had: 'I can do this… I can do more than I think I can.' Over the next couple of months she joined me in a few other locations, upping her distance each time and running further than she'd ever run before. Then she ran her first marathon with me in Liverpool, a year to the day since she started running. Being part of that was so memorable. Her journey related so much to mine, and we've shared something very special. It's one of the major memories of the challenge.

And what about afterwards? I catch up with Ben a few months later, just after he's set up his new 401 Foundation. It's terrific to find him so well and happy, but it's been a bit of a rocky road getting there.

At the end of the challenge, there was a bit of a void. I needed to find my new purpose, and my new sense of normal. And because I put my body through such a physiological trauma, my serotonin levels were depleted because I was adrenaline-focused right the way through. Actually I fell into a state of depression after the project. I didn't sleep for two months. Every time I went to bed, I'd lie down and my heart rate would jump to about 180 beats a minute. The adrenaline would course through my body and I'd be wide awake and stressing about the fact that I was self employed. I needed to create a new life, to find out what the new thing was going to be.

The awards we received through that period of depression were amazing. I was having such high highs. But for instance, the morning of Sports Personality of the Year I was on the sofa crying my eyes out to Kyle, my partner, saying, 'I can't do this. I just can't function.'

We have a new direction now, which is The 401 Foundation. It's the legacy. A grant-based foundation that will support grass-roots projects throughout the UK. They build confidence and self-esteem, but obviously tackle mental health and self-development issues. That, twinned with all the motivational speaking that I seem to be doing around the country, it's a busy, but a happy life. A life that I chose and a life that I created for myself. Not one that I've fitted myself into.

And as for my Sunday morning jaunt straight after running around the Isle of Wight? I think the word ponderous is probably best to describe it. With a dash of laborious and a hint of overdoing it. I was thrilled when the family got home.

17. wendover

'This is a bit like the Barkley Marathons,' says a fellow runner as we both puff up another surprisingly spiteful hill in a wood just north of London.

It is of course *nothing at all* like the Barkley Marathons, that notoriously brutal, idiosyncratic 100(ish)-miler in the mountains of Tennessee. The one with the 1% finish rate. For a start this race is just 50 miles long, and instead of the wilds of the Crab Orchard Mountains, it's being staged (for the very first time as it happens) in a relatively small area of woodland near the market town of Wendover in the Chiltern Hills. Children come here to play; by the side of the path, about a mile into the race, there's a wood carving of a Gruffalo. Central London is less than an hour away. The route is well marked and marshalled so nobody gets lost. There's an aid station every five miles. And nobody's playing 'The Last Post' on a bugle every time a runner drops out.

And yet, I sort of know what she means. For a start, we're running five loops like they do in Tennessee. And some of these uphills are genuinely nasty. I'm flailing upwards like a baby giraffe learning to walk and wishing I'd brought poles. Also, as this race is brand new – we're in the middle of lap one of the inaugural Wendover Woods 50 – nobody really knows where we're going.

This is James Elson's newest race. You'll remember James from the SDW100 and thinking back on it now, he did warn me about the Wendover hills in an email: 'There are climbs on this course which are steep in anyone's book. We wanted to include features you can reflect on and explain to your mates how epic they were. You may need to use trees as resting posts. Runners have returned from recces with reports of unrunnable bushwhacking. The course is tough. No doubt.' So tough in fact, that James has had to increase the time limit from 13 hours, which is usual at his 50-milers, to 16 hours. He's also named the hills: one of them's called 'Boulevard of Broken Dreams'. And there was me thinking he was a nice guy!

This fiendish new race looks to be as popular as all the others. There are people moaning about these hills, but only in that endurance runner way when they're actually quite enjoying the challenge. It seems, even so early in the race, that the Wendover Woods 50 can be declared a success and will stick around on the calendar. But what about the future, both for James and the sport in the UK?

I've got a few ideas for events I'd like to add. None of them fits really into the template of what we're currently doing. The things that have crossed my mind are a 50km or some kind of entry-level ultra distance – somewhere between the marathon and the 50-milers because that's a big jump. And there's a huge demand for that.

Also a 24-hour track event. And a very hard mountain 100 in the UK – a Lakeland 100 that goes over all the tops rather than the Lakeland 100 course that avoids them. However, the major issue with something like that is you're badly stepping on somebody else's toes.

And we've had people do that to us. We had an event a couple of years ago, they tried to organise a South Downs 100 starting at Chilcomb exactly where we begin ours and finishing at the rugby ground next to our track, using the same checkpoint locations. I didn't say anything, I just let them do their thing. And as it turned out, nobody supported the event, they didn't get any entries and it died out. I think people immediately saw that it was just a copy, a literal exact copy, of something that's being done perfectly well elsewhere.

So these things have to be done with a level of observation of what other people are doing.

Now in five years' time, we could have another 15-, 20,000 ultra-runners, which is probably the rate of growth from the last five years. In which case a vast array of new opportunities opens up for people. That's great, if it happens. But I worry that one big operator could come in and suck so much life out of the rest of the sport that everyone else struggles.

Right now, there are people with struggles of a different kind. We're on the fifth significant climb of this first of five laps, and wondering how much more punishment there's still to come.

In my case, it doesn't help that I'm still sick. I've had a low-level illness ever since I returned to running too soon after the South Downs Way 100. James himself did warn me against it. But two days after crossing the finishing line, my legs seemed OK, so I experimented with a gentle run to work. That went well, so I ran home again a little harder. By the Thursday, I was back in full training mode, thrilled that my legs had decided to work again so soon.

It was a month before I noticed any problem. I learned, too late, that your endocrine (glandular) system takes longer to recover from running 100 miles than your mind or your legs. A deep kind of lethargy set in, both in myself and my running pace. I just felt a tiny bit poorly, constantly. Like I was at the very start or the very end of a cold. It wasn't severe enough to stop me doing anything – but everything I did, especially any exercise, was underwhelming.

It all came to a head during the New York Marathon, which I'd trained hard for. Terrific race, brilliant atmosphere and a real sense of a journey through the five distinct boroughs. But I didn't enjoy any of it. I ran flat out, but was 20 full minutes slower than I'd hoped for. And I promptly got properly sick, a kidney infection, which I'm still suffering aftershocks from in Wendover.

Mind you, following the New York Marathon with a 50-mile race an hour from your front door is nothing. Jules Hall and I became pals when he was part of our BBC Children in Need team in the Big Apple. He finished three minutes ahead of me in Central Park. His next stop was the vast emptiness of Arctic Canada for the frankly terrifying 430-mile Montane Yukon Arctic Ultra. Temperatures can drop to −40 degrees, plus wind chill.

It's twice as cold as your freezer. You get out there and your eyebrows and your eyes start freezing instantly and you're thinking, 'This is just not right.' It freaks you out. You can't train to be that cold, you just have to accept it. I'm keyed up for the race, I've done the training, I'm here, I'm going to give it my best shot.

Then the race briefing is the part where they tell you everything that can possibly go wrong. So they're telling you all the dangers of frostbite, dehydration, falling through the ice. In that environment you can be up to 24 hours from any help. It's unbelievably cold. They can't just send a helicopter to pick you up. They have to get Skidoos out and the Skidoos have to drive maybe 70 miles to come and get you and sometimes the Skidoos don't start.

So they give you a dressing down; they tell you this is serious. And that's the point when you start thinking, 'This is not such a great idea.' Then you have the bit where people ask questions, but in my head I was going, 'Shut up, I just don't want to know.' I remember someone saying, 'What about wolves? What about bears?' And they said, 'Well, it would be very early for a bear to come out of hibernation.' And you're like, 'Don't tell me that, just tell me it's asleep until the summer. I'd rather not know.' They're warning you that one of the things to be scared of is moose. The moose are very big and very dumb so if you're walking down the trail and if a moose is walking the other way, you think you'll nip into the trees and go around, but he'll think there's someone on his trail and charge you. And if you've got a one-tonne moose heading at you then what do you do?

That briefing was a chance to get properly scared, then you've got a day or two to sort your kit out, pack everything, check it, re-check it. Because once you're out the door, if you've left something, say a pair of gloves, it's curtains.

The whole race follows the Yukon quest, retracing the steps of this old supply route for the gold rush. 430 miles from Whitehorse to Dawson City. By the first aid station I was freezing, hypothermic. They give you some food, generally a frozen sandwich, and you go again.

The first aid station is shocking. People on the bed shaking. They're so weak, their lungs have packed up and they can't breathe properly. Within two days, half the field dropped out. One guy, the first night, went to put up his tent, took off his gloves and put his hand on the pole. His hand froze solid to the pole and that's him out of the race.

The worst thing is when you're at the aid station where there's a fire, just some warmth, you've got to motivate yourself to go back into the cold, into the middle of nowhere for another 50 or 70 miles.

It's best if you run from four or five in the morning right through to one or two in the morning, get whatever sleep you can and then set off. Best to keep moving and keep warm. When you stop, that's when you get really cold. So beforehand you're thinking about how to get my tent up, how to get in there, what do I need to bring with me, where's the stuff in my sled.

You get in the sleeping bag as quickly as possible, you fall asleep because you're just so tired but then half an hour later you wake up because it's so cold your body's checking if you're still alive. You're desperate for it to get light because it's so cold, it's just so horrible.

When you get into your sleeping bag at night, you put your shoes in with you, take your water pack off and everything goes in the sleeping bag with you to stop it freezing. Anything you leave out for 10 minutes will freeze. You don't want to be putting on frozen shoes in the morning.

At one point I thought I was going to have to drop out because of chafing. The whole time you're eating frozen sweets or frozen meat. You're 50 miles from the next checkpoint, you don't see anyone for that whole period of time, you're tired, your mind's asking 'Why am I doing this? Is it worth continuing?'

There was one guy, an experienced ultra-runner, he thought he was being followed by a pack of wolves for two days. And he dropped out of the race because basically he freaked out. And I heard about this and I thought, 'That's a bit weak'. But to hear him speak about it, you completely understand. You're in that environment, you're cold, you're tired, you're not thinking straight. You look behind you and you see a pair of eyes. Then you see a pair of eyes in front of you. In the cold light of day, if you look at it dispassionately and statistically, you know you're pretty safe and they'll eventually disappear.

But at night you see shadows. You start to hallucinate. You see stuff in the trees. All you've got is your torch beam and all you ever see anywhere is snow and trees. And then you see something in the trees and you're not quite sure what it is. And you just do that thing where you close your eyes and you say whatever it was, I don't care, just keep ploughing forward.

At 300 miles I thought, what's the difference between a 300-mile Arctic ultra and 430? What am I trying to prove here? But I did the race for a mental health charity called Place2Be, who help kids in schools if they're depressed or being bullied. That was one thing that kept me going. The other thing was I've done a few of these races, and I just thought once I've done this, I'm done. I've got nothing left to prove.

When you cross the finish line, you're 50% dead, but the most elated you've ever been because you've just done something that no one else will get to experience. That is the most life-affirming sensation – you've just completed something that has put you right on the edge of what it means to be alive. It's this unique feeling, almost floating. A mixture of pure elation, utter exhaustion, and I got so lonely, so very lonely. I've never missed my family so much.

But I'm a way better person for doing what I do. Endurance running, I think for certain people, it's like the perfect drug in that it puts you physically and mentally in great condition. I've got a reasonably stressful job and I'm able to cope with so much more. The results of running every day and having these goals and having something else to worry about other than the day-to-day. You free up your brain from anxiety and stress.

And actually, it teaches you so much that's valuable for life, self-confidence, resilience, the ability to stick through things when they're tough going.

Back in Wendover, I'm finding this 50-mile race just about exactly tough enough to get the benefits Jules was talking about. Some of them at least. The hills are sharp enough to be approached with apprehension, and I'm feeling under the weather. I run past my car, and the temptation to get in and drive home – well it's not exactly overwhelming, but it's certainly present.

But I'm also discovering that there's something quite appealing about running laps. By the third time around, you know the course pretty well and are prepared for what's coming. Perhaps this is how runners who recce race routes feel all the time. It's both comforting and intimidating. You can also accurately measure your physical deterioration by seeing how much longer every lap takes. I only manage the first 10 miles in reasonably good order before basically capitulating. The second and third are difficult. Throughout most of the fourth loop, I'm convinced I won't run a fifth. But I do. And enjoy it.

A head torch is part of the mandatory kit for this race, but I didn't imagine I'd need it. An 8am start time in late November gives over eight hours of daylight, easily enough time, I reckoned, as I packed my kit before dawn trying not to wake the children again, to finish before dusk. I reckoned without the hills and my illness. In fact only the first two runners cover the 50 miles in under eight hours. The rest of us need torches.

Only mine's low on power and the light it's emitting is barely worthy of the name. I do have some spare batteries – again, they're compulsory – but I'm sure they're old. So sure that I don't even bother to check. Instead, in the pitch blackness of the woods, I learn a new skill – light-borrowing. What you do is speed up or slow down until you're with your nearest fellow runner, then fall in behind them and run at their pace. It helps if you ask first. When you sense that he or she is getting tired of your heavy breathing in their ear, or if you're struggling to keep up, you move on to the next competitor with a working torch. Another advantage of a looped course: there's always someone quite close by.

My wife calls. A working mobile phone is also on the kit list. She's come to surprise me with the kids but they just missed me at the 40-mile start/finish area. There's no chance of hooking up later in the course so I offer to run back the mile-and-a-half to see them. Obviously I'm expecting them to gracefully refuse – I've just run 42 miles after all. So I'm ever so slightly miffed when they accept. I grumble and grouse whilst retracing my steps, but by the time I see them I both look, and am, genuinely delighted. Though I'm definitely keen to get going again after a quick hug, if for no other reason than it's absolutely freezing when you stop running.

The four of them head back into the nice warm car with its comfy, heated seats, and cheerfully describe how they've found a fabulous Italian restaurant for dinner. So while I tackle those hills one final time, all the while I'm fantasising about spaghetti.

I make do with a petrol station snack on the way home, a Scotch egg on the very edge of its use by date. But it's been another terrific day on the trail and I feel extremely fortunate to be able to run and enjoy events like this. And I treasure my post-race photo. It's framed on the mantelpiece at home (and also quite prominent on the WW50 website). My elder kids are in it, grinning as widely as I am and showing my medal to the camera. Honestly, crossing a finishing line with your children; you really can't beat it.

18. sparta

Still 20-odd miles to go on the road to Sparta when I suffer a catastrophic loss of leg power. It's the only way to describe it. And it's significantly sub-optimal when you've almost a marathon still to run and time is not your friend. Actually, there's quite a long list of things that are currently not my friend. Time and my trashed legs being the top two. But also in the top five: my stomach, which feels like it's hosting a war; my feet (I dread to think what they look like, I'm just aware of constant pain and a strange liquid sensation inside my socks); and my brain – somebody's superglued my synapses.

I've had no sleep in almost 30 hours, and just three hours' sleep in 50. In my job I'm used to early starts and busy days on little sleep, so I naively thought I'd cope with the sleep deprivation side of this Greek adventure. I thought wrong! I attempt to work out what speed I need to travel to make it to the finish in time. This is crucial information but the maths, so easy a few miles ago, seems too daunting to even contemplate now. I need something easier to get the grey matter working, a squat for the mind. How about simply how far is there to go? Everything is in kilometres here, and I know the race is just under 247. So... I've already run about 220km, which means... hang on... 247km plus... no, minus... no, I was right first time, 247 plus... or is it minus...? I must make a funny sight, legs shuffling, eyes squinting in concentration.

Casting my mind back now, only a few weeks afterwards, I only have vague recollections of the hours that followed, snippets of memory. Like the morning after a particularly boozy night, trying to piece together what happened through the foggy backwaters of the mind. Only without the nagging dread of 'did I make a fool of myself?'

Some things I do remember:

Cars and lorries drive past in both directions and almost every one of them hoots in support. I begin to fear the sound of an engine. Raising an arm to acknowledge the encouragement is using energy I simply don't have at my disposal. I try to smile but suspect it looks more like a grimace.

At one particular checkpoint, it must be the one with 24km to go, I recall a friendly volunteer telling me I've done it. *Only a half-marathon to go!* he chirps. *Give or take. And most of it is gently downhill on a smooth road. How long can that take – two hours? Two-and-a-half?*

I'd been looking forward to the final half-marathon. I'd been convinced I'd find the strength to run strong for the final 13 miles, but I'd reckoned without whatever's happened to most of my muscles below the waist. All I can do is move forwards as quickly as the shattered, pulverised legs will carry me, which – trust me – is an awful lot slower than two-and-a-half-hour half-marathon pace.

One thing I'm strongly aware of, is the fact that I'm not stopping. I had my mental wobble at dawn and I came through it. The only way I'm failing to reach the statue is if I literally collapse (which is a proper possibility) or I fail to make one of the cut-offs (also a clear and present danger).

A memory pops unexpectedly into my head from the bus ride to the Acropolis. A conversation with my roommate Mick, who I sincerely hope will have finished by now.

'What are you hoping for, Mick, if everything goes according to plan? Do you have a time or position in mind?'

'Well I definitely want to finish in less than 30 hours. Definitely. And as for position, we'll see. It would be nice to be overtaking people at the end. How about you, what if everything goes right?'

I remember how the question surprised me because I'd never previously considered the possibility of something major not going wrong. Eventually I came up with:

'I'd like to have built enough of a time buffer so I don't have to be stressed at the end. To have, say, three hours for the final half-marathon so I just know for certain I'm going to make it to the statue in time. Then I can relax and enjoy the end of the journey.'

That was my perfect scenario. The way it's worked out – well let's call it a partial success. On the one hand, I have a significantly bigger buffer than three hours. But there's definitely no relaxing and enjoying the journey. I'm constantly having to move forwards as fast as I can. Breaking down the fibres of the muscles one by one with every footstep, leaving fewer functioning fibres for the next one. At some point I fear I'll simply run out of fibres. I'm desperately trying to bank the miles whilst I'm able, ticking them off one by one before the legs stop working completely and I have to start crawling.

It never quite comes to that, but it's not far off.

Some other random recollections.

First seeing Sparta, a sprawling collection of white buildings and orange roofs. It looks glorious in sunshine, surrounded by green olive trees and grey mountains. Less than six miles to go now, not even a 10K. However, setting eyes on the town for the first time makes getting there somehow less likely. Sparta looks impossibly far away, nestling in the valley away to our right. And then the road promptly veers left. I shiver despite the heat of the day. This is a long way from done.

I'm being overtaken frequently; it's long since lost its sting. This is not a race against others, it's about finding a way to reach the finishing line. This is me versus me. Some runners slow to ask if they can help but most do not – it's become attritional for everyone. There are just so many things that can go badly wrong in a race as long as 153 miles. Almost all of us will have suffered at least one calamity along the way. And despite the fact that I'm barely moving forward and have the arthritic gait of a dying giraffe, I count myself among the lucky ones.

Then with 5km to go, the shining thought bursts through that I'll finish. I have enough time, if needs be, to crawl to the statue from here. Tears bristle the corners of my eyes. These ones aren't salty. These are happy tears.

There's typical Greek chaos surrounding the penultimate checkpoint. There are cars everywhere, drivers attempting ridiculous manoeuvres on the busy road, yet still no angry horns. The only hoots are honks of support for the runners (I'm using the term 'runner' very loosely by now). Then, from the back window of a taxi attempting the most ludicrous U-turn I've ever seen, two voices I recognise. My brilliant dad and wonderful step-mother Annie. They've been in the Peloponnese all week, arranged the trip especially to meet me at the finish and experience Sparta on Spartathlon Saturday. It's amazing to see them, even as my dad causes further traffic turmoil by opening the door of the taxi to give me a kiss and say hello.

'How are you doing, Vassos?'

'Terrible! But never happier.'

'You've done great. See you in Sparti*.'

'Yep, see you in Sparti. Thank you. I may be a while yet though.'

It takes over an hour to negotiate those final five kilometres. I have no idea what happened for 2.6 of them, but I'll remember the final 2.4km forever.

As you complete the Spartathlon, you cross the River Eurotas on the outskirts of the town. There's a sign welcoming you to Sparta and a checkpoint with a timing mat by the side of the road. For the past 150-plus miles, there have only been half a dozen timing mats at most, so for a moment you think 'This is it, I've done it. I've reached Sparta, so this timing mat must be the final destination. Where's King Leonidas?' But then the volunteers cheerfully tell you – they genuinely believe they're delivering good news – that there are 2.4km remaining. I happen to know that's exactly a mile-and-a-half, and I almost give up for the second time. The thought of another mile-and-a-half seems unbearable.

However, several kids, random local kids, some on bikes and some on foot, come to my rescue. Before my nascent sulk has a chance to grow into anything ugly, a boy of about 10 takes my hand and begins walking with me into the town. As soon as it emerges that I'm Greek,

---

* The town of Sparta is now known as Sparti in Greek. In the 1830s King Otto ordered the construction of a new Sparta to honour its ancient glory. Sparti was the first town in Greece to be constructed to an architectural plan.

more kids appear. We start chatting about running generally, and my new friend tells me proudly how he recently completed his first 10K.

A much younger child pipes up. He's been desperate to say something but now he has my attention, he seems to struggle to find the words. Eventually he works it out.

'Why are you going so... slowly?' he demands.

'Ha! I've just run from Athens and it's honestly not nearby.'

'Yeah, but still...'

'Yeah, well – sorry!'

'So hurry up!'

'Can't!'

'Can!'

'Honestly, I can't.'

'Honestly, at least try....'

It's one of my favourite ever conversations.

Every time we pass a building, people on balconies stand to applaud. Soon we're into the centre of the town where cheering pedestrians line the streets. I finish at lunchtime and every roadside taverna is full. As I stagger past, the diners interrupt their meals to stand up and clap. This isn't like a big city marathon where there's a constant stream of runners to keep you interested. Here there were only 400 of us to start with. The lucky few who reach Sparta – it's around half this year, unusually high – are spread over 12 hours. So you can go a long time without seeing a finisher. But each of us is treated to the same warmth of welcome.

Through the town and I'm lapping up the atmosphere, drinking in every sight and sound. A part of me wishes I could muster a run, it would seem befitting, but I know that's impossible. We turn right up and up a hill. There are even more people on this street, more cheers, more applause. It's wonderful.

Leonidas was not the King of Sparta when Pheidippides completed his epic journey in 490BC. He was in charge a decade later, when the Persians arrived for a second try. Known as the warrior king, Leonidas led a tiny force of elite troops, immortalised in the film *300*, at the Battle of Thermopylae. The Spartan 300 were outnumbered by a thousand to one. The enormous statue in Sparta has an inscription on the plinth that reads 'MOLON LABE' ('Come and take them'). This was Leonidas' reply when Xerxes, the Persian ruler, offered to spare Spartan lives if they gave up their arms.

Another right turn (have we doubled back on ourselves?) and suddenly the statue is visible through a forest of flags. I launch one final, monumental effort to force a run, and practically fall over. I resolve instead to enjoy the moment for all it's worth. The atmosphere throughout the race has been second to none. The volunteers have been amazing. Everything has worked perfectly. And the climax in Sparta is all I could have hoped for and more. Like I said at the start, this is not just another race. You're not running an arbitrary number of miles from one place to another or around in a circle. You're recreating one of the most important ancient endurance runs in history and especially here in Greece, that really means something. With every footstep towards the statue, I feel increasingly anchored to a glorious past.

But now there are four stairs to climb. On legs which no longer bend. There are people all around, crowds thronging the finish area. The guy on the microphone is introducing me on the PA system. 'This man is Greek,' he's saying. 'He's called Vassos and he lives in London. But he's Greek.' This goes down well with the locals. They love a home finisher.

There's just a moment, no longer than a second, when I fear I'm going to disgrace myself and be forced to crawl up to the statue. But somehow I manage it on two legs. Climb the steps. Raise my arms. Kiss the foot.

It's done.

And it's the best feeling ever.

Local young people dressed in ancient costumes offer me water from the River Eurotas in a stone goblet, just like Pheidippides would have been given 2,500 years earlier. An olive wreath is placed on my head, a small trophy handed to me along with a neon yellow 'Spartathlon Finisher' T-shirt. A truly appalling colour. My first thought is 'I'll never wear *that*'. But as it happens, like New Yorkers who complete their home marathon and proudly wear the medal for days, I'll rarely remove the T-shirt for the next month.

I'm ushered straight into the medical tent after finishing. It looks like something out of a Vietnam War film. Patients lying semi-conscious hooked up to intravenous drips, others shivering, some convulsing. And the state of their feet... All told it seems I escaped quite lightly. And with memories to last a lifetime.

19. alabama

The Spartathlon was my Everest. Beforehand, if you'd offered me the option to complete the race but injure myself so badly I wouldn't run for six months, I'd have probably taken it. But now... well I've had my cake and eaten it, completed the Spartathlon without doing myself any serious damage... now I get to start contemplating the next cake.

For around 40 hours after kissing the statue in Sparta, I can't move my legs. Or rather, I can only move my legs if I use my arms to do so. The only physical way I'm able to get either leg from one position to another is to shove them there. Otherwise the legs just follow me limply about, attached by the waist but utterly incapable of independent action. I haul myself where I need to go.

On that first night, I flop onto the mattress with my legs hanging over the side. And that's how I stay, sleeping in the shape of a twisted right angle. The prospect of having to sit up and somehow force the legs into a position where they're not making my lower back ache is worse than the actual ache. I'm thankful that I'm too dehydrated to need the loo.

The following day there are celebrations planned in Sparta. However I have to fly home, back to work on Monday morning, plus I don't like being away from Caroline and the kids a moment longer than necessary. I was of course sorry to be missing the formal Sunday lunch hosted by the mayor, and indeed the gala dinner in Athens the following evening. But as I wake in the morning, it occurs to me that even if I were staying in Greece, I'd be unable to attend. How on earth would I get there? My legs have become nothing but burdens.

I muster all my little remaining energy and crawl commando-style to the bathroom, slither over the edge of the bath and lower myself into the water head first. Groaning constantly. It takes an hour to get washed and dressed, and I'm proud I manage it so quickly.

I need wheelchairs to get me through the airports. After we land back in London, a friendly Jordanian meets me off the plane and pushes me through passport control and out into the Heathrow arrivals hall. My children are somewhat taken aback to see me so incapacitated. I suspect my wife is too, but she's better at hiding it. For my part, I've never been happier to see them.

We head straight to our local hospital where they lend me a Zimmer frame to get about. Gradually, over the next few days, life begins seeping back into my legs.

Meanwhile, goodness knows what I'm sweating out the other way. I spend the first week sleeping on the sofa (a staircase being a challenge too far) and awake every morning with the cushions soaking wet. I try turning them over but the sweat has gone right through. It's kind of cool and simultaneously absolutely gross. We end up having to buy a new sofa.

And it's whilst researching the sofa purchase online, that my mind starts wandering to future running events. It's been ages since I didn't have a big challenge in the diary – the possibilities are wonderfully diverse. My browser search history changes from 'London sofa shops' to 'worldwide ultra-marathons'.

Previously I'd been considering the possibility of mounting one final assault on the road marathon PB. My friend Nick from the 50-mile Mendip Marauder race went straight on to the Bournemouth Marathon and was buzzing after achieving a lifetime best and winning his age group. I've been wondering whether with six months' dedicated training, I could cajole my marathon time under 2:50.

Several pals from Barnes Runners have been mildly obsessed with their marathon times ever since I've known them. And when I say 'mildly' I mean 'completely'. Minutes after crossing the finishing line in London, they booked into the Valencia marathon. (I admit to being part of this lunacy. Those who subsequently broke three hours in the Spanish city have been referring to themselves as the Sub-3 Amigos.) I've never trained for a marathon with a running club before. I could simply dive in to the Tuesday tempos and Thursday track sessions and see how much I can shave off the PB. I'm in my early forties, I won't get many more chances.

And yet.

Do I really care anymore? Training for and achieving a desired time can be enormously rewarding. For ages, my Holy Grail was a marathon time starting with a '2'. Pulling that off remains one of my proudest moments. But the journey as a whole, whilst satisfying and eventful, was never especially joyful. Definitely not the training, and not many of the races either.

Running on the trail on the other hand... multi-day mountain races, a Bob Graham Round... I'm whizzing through the options like a kid in a sweet shop. The Comrades Marathon in South Africa must be high on the list, just for its sheer history and scale. And also one of the iconic American 100-milers. I've heard amazing tales of Western States, Hardrock 100, Leadville....

Nobody has won more of these than Karl Meltzer, 'Speedgoat Karl.' I catch up with him a few days before his 39th victory over 100 miles, and then again 48 hours after he leads home the field on the Pinhoti Trail in Alabama. Karl has now won at least one 100-mile race a year for a remarkable 17 years. His motto is, '*100 miles is not that far*'.

I've been ultra-running for 20 years, and the scene has changed a lot, mostly because of social media. But in general to me, it still feels the same. I'm still alone running in the woods daily, and at races, what can be better than that?

I'll tell you what I love most about it... Just the serenity of being in the mountains or woods, running alone or being supported. And at the same time, it's a race. I like the strategy behind longer races as it's not all about speed. Strategy is important, and I like to outwit people by running smart. I never really liked fast, hard races, but the longer ones are easier because we are not suffering as much cardio-wise.

Plus it always feels great to complete a long run. That feeling definitely intensifies with longer distances. I really don't get warmed up until about mile 40-ish, where I find my zone.

Then it's all fun and sometimes pain from there, but the satisfaction of completing it always makes it worthwhile. To get through the tough times, music is my go to. I always tell myself how lucky I am to be a pro runner. Any real athlete would say that, it's an honour to do what I do. So stop complaining.

Thing is though, when you're the legs underneath Karl Meltzer, there's plenty of cause for complaint. They once propelled him to six 100-mile race victories in a single year, most in record time, and the final four all within a frenetic eight-week period. Mere mortals take months to recover from running these distances – and as I know to my cost, rushing back can be counterproductive. So I find myself asking Karl how long it takes his mind and body to bounce back from a 100-miler, and if there's anything he does to help speed up the process.

Depends. It takes me up to five weeks usually, based on what kind of shape I was in at the start. But I come back slow and never push training too quickly. If I run lots of 100s within a few weeks, I don't run long runs in between. I let feel be my method of recovery, not a 'schedule'.

I have always worked to live, never lived to work. And in running, I've done exactly that. It's what I do, and I refuse to let others dictate my life, even if I may not be a perfect role model. I have no fears for the future, we all get older. I just want to keep running, regardless of pace.

That final sentence resonates. *I just want to keep running, regardless of pace.* It's how I feel too. The marathon PB can stay where it is for the moment. Especially as, hot on the heels of Speedgoat Karl, I get to talk to another of the greats to the US ultra scene. Charlie Engle has been winning races and completing amazing challenges since the 1980s.

He was deeply hungover for his very first endurance run, the Big Sur Marathon of 1989. He'd been on the drink and drugs until the early hours of race day and only just made it back to his hotel room to change before boarding the 5:30am bus to the start. Four miles from the finish he necked two cans of lager, hair of the dog. As soon as he got home, he called his drug dealer. Fair to say Charlie's come a long way since.

I am a recovering addict with 25 years clean and sober, but just because I'm sober doesn't mean I don't like to continue to take risks. And one of the things that ultra-running does for me is to allow me, in a sort of controlled environment, to put myself in a position where, even if the physical risks are not huge, I think the emotional risks are great. I've never stepped onto the start line of a 100-miler and thought, 'Oh, this is going to be easy'. And that's what I love about it.

I did a lot of marathons for years and I reached a point where I felt absolutely certain I was going to finish. And I missed that edginess and uncertainty that came with doing something that I wasn't sure that I could actually do.

It's what continues to this day to lead me to find longer and different challenges out of my comfort zone. But the ultra-distance is necessary for me because, as I like to say, in a 100-miler it takes the first marathon just to scrape away that scuzzy top layer that I carry around all the time and get down to the good stuff, the cool, clear water underneath. And I think it offers me some relief, in a way, from daily life but also a better glimpse of myself and of the underlying motivations for not just my athletic stuff but for the rest of my life.

I'm not sure I ever feel true joy when I finish an event because, frankly, in most cases, I planned and trained and worked really hard to get there, whether it's an event of someone else's making or a self-made adventure. And while there's satisfaction, there's something sad about being done with a big project. Finishing my run across the Sahara Desert and putting my feet in the Red Sea was one of the saddest moments of my life because I knew there was no going back. I knew

I could never go back and have those exact experiences again. It may sound like a cliché, but it's true. It genuinely is the journey and not the finish line that is most important.

I will tell you another insight I think you would find interesting and probably not surprising. The ultra-world in general is loaded with addicts, recovering or not. And I mean the term addict in a very general sense.

Charlie once ran across America in a relay team of six to heighten awareness of mental illness. Six runners with a history of mental illness running 3100 miles, 5 million footsteps, with a message of hope for those suffering from depression, addiction and other disorders. Running for – not from – mental illness.

And it worked. The mental health landscape has changed significantly in recent years, almost entirely for the better, and sport and sportspeople can take much of the credit. At the 2017 London Marathon, the official charity was Heads Together, a mental health charity set up by the Duke and Duchess of Cambridge and Prince Harry. Tens of thousands of people ran through the streets of London wearing headbands to help tackle the stigma that prevents people from talking about issues or getting help. Prince William said it was 'time for Britain to abandon its stiff upper lip'.

The endurance running scene in the USA is following a similar trajectory. These days, you tell people you're running 100 miles and it's kind of no big deal. And that's a massive change since Charlie started running in the 1980s, when a half marathon was epic. So what are his hopes and fears for his chosen sport in the future?

It's fascinating to me to have watched the sport change because I have been at it for decades. I'm 55 years old but even now, and certainly in my forties, I could be competitive with the best in the world. And even beat most of them some of the time. I like to say that for ultra-distance sports you need to have been alive long enough to learn how to suffer.

As it turns out that's no longer true. There are still tons of people of my age in the sport, but there's been a real shift. There are now a lot of 20-somethings getting into it. And quite frankly, they're skipping the marathon altogether. I know people who have never run a marathon but they're winning 100-mile races.

Years ago I spoke at a marathon in Des Moines, Iowa. I was speaking to an audience of 500 people the night before and I narrowed them down to this one 18-year-old who was running his first marathon the next day. I said, 'It's your first marathon. Are you nervous?' I handed him the microphone. He's like, 'No, I ran a 50-miler last month.' And I said, 'So what made you do that? Why would you start with a 50-miler?' And, totally straight-faced, he took the mic back and replied: 'Dude, my mom ran a marathon.'

He wasn't being diminishing of the marathon, but young people want to be different. Marathoning specifically is still fantastic. And I still think it's one of the hardest things there is to do. If I toe the line in a marathon with the aim of running my fastest time, whatever that might be on the day, it's going to hurt like hell. Ultras, for whatever reason, have now attracted these young people who are just doing crazy things and they're amazing. They're good for the sport. Records are falling all over the place. I'm sure the same thing is happening in the UK. It's just fascinating to see this shift. And in the social media world we live in, I think a lot of it is driven by a need to both be different, and look different. And I love the attitude that people don't want to just follow the same path as their predecessors.

However, I read some articles recently about races that are now having trouble filling their rosters. I live in North Carolina, and 10 years ago there might have been half a dozen ultra-distance races in the state. Today there's half a dozen every weekend. Which is great for convenience. It's not great for the level of competition.

So I think we've reached this point where probably, very much like marathoning too, I think we'll see a lot of the smaller races begin to disappear. Which isn't necessarily a good thing but I think that it does help strengthen the stronger races.

Ultra-running needs to be careful not to make the big events so elite there are only a few people who can get in. I love Badwater for that reason. The race director there, Chris Kostman, mandates that 50% of his field every single year is new people. As long as you meet the qualification criteria: a minimum of three 100-milers. But half the people in the race are new to the race. I love that attitude and I would like to see a lot of the other big races, even the lottery races, do that same thing somehow. Make sure places are filled by people who are relatively new to the sport so we can keep the excitement going.

I don't think running is going anywhere though. I think marathoning and ultra-running will continue to grow. Personally, I'm always looking for the next big adventure. I think as long as people continue to look for new and exciting places in the world to run, I think the sport will continue to grow.

I hope he's right, because there's still so much I want to experience. Part of me wishes I'd discovered endurance running a decade ago. Being at the vanguard of a sport growing exponentially must have been truly exhilarating. A little like the UK triathletes in the early 2000s when the sport had recently made its Olympic debut in Sydney.

Endurance running still has some way to go to catch up with triathlon in popularity, but it's on a similar curve. It's still an exciting place to be.

I wonder how soon it'll be before people don't bat an eyelid when you tell them you're running 100 miles in one go. Forty years ago, only 'lunatics' ran marathons.

20. why

When you run silly distances, the question of 'why' pops up a lot. Why bother? Why run for five hours when you could stay in shape in 20 minutes? Why push yourself to extremes? Why isn't a marathon enough?

Why choose a sport in which blisters are a badge of honour and suffering is mandatory? Why, when there's little prize money on offer (and usually none at all)? Why, when even the very best endurance runners are little-known and most have to work proper jobs just to get by? Why, when training alone requires many hours alone on the trail.

Why aren't you normal?

That's the thing really, isn't it? That final question, that's the heart of the matter. Are we really 'mad' like so many people seem to suggest?

A morning on the Breakfast Show – three hours of barely moving in a radio studio – followed by another two hours behind the wheel of a car driving north. By the time I reach my friend Claire's house, I'm pulling my hair out. I just need to *move!*

Fortunately, Claire happens to be my guru in all things trail running and before we even have a cup of tea, she's leading me out on a run. First through the town she's just moved into – recently voted the best place to live in the UK with its 17th-century stone buildings and medieval churches – and then, blissfully, through a muddy field, into some woods, up a hill....

For a while we stop chatting and just enjoy the glorious views, soak up our surroundings, concentrate on not losing our footing. The absorption is deeply consuming. We both lose ourselves and soon find ourselves refreshed.

The Japanese call it Shinrin-Yoku, or 'forest bathing'. Simply visit a natural area and enjoy all sorts of calming, rejuvenating and restorative benefits. It's a cornerstone of Japanese healthcare. Running too has been proven to offer numerous physical and mental health enhancements. Combine the two and – bingo!

'I think as human beings we just forgot that this is what we need to do.' This is Claire Maxted when I ask her for her thoughts over a delicious lunchtime salad. For many years she was the editor of *Trail Running* magazine before setting up on her own as Wild Ginger Films. She definitely knows her stuff.

The anxiety problems and increasing levels of depression and mental health issues in our society come from us having lost our roots – rather than humans just having these problems anyway, and then addressing them with the running. I think it's the other way around. I think we dropped the running and the physical exercise, and we got these problems as a result. And now we've discovered that we need to hit the trails.

I think running for a long time, say four or five or even six hours is an excuse to get away and be free. You can't really check your phone or your emails. Just enjoy the experience, talk to people, meet new people, be in the moment. One of the best races I've been on, the Coastal Challenge across Costa Rica, all you had to do was run, pack your bag, eat, run, try not to stop, try to ignore the pain and the blisters, and then chat with other nice people, eat nice food, sleep, pack your bag, and get up and run again the next day. It's a very simple life on some of these multi-day events and ultra-races. Lots of food, sweets, chatting and running around. Basically, it's a moving party.

I do think more and more people are realising the need to connect with nature and to move. Because all jobs used to be quite manual and full-on, certainly for men, while women were attending the house, doing the housework, doing the chores, moving all the time. But now more and more of us are in offices, just literally sitting. It's just not enough.

For me, I know that I need to breathe, and breathe deeply, because otherwise I spin off into various stages of anxiety or excitement that are uncontrollable. So, running is a form of moving yoga for me, and I just have to get out there. A sort of a meditation and exercise all in one. Otherwise I feel trapped in a cage. That's honestly how I feel. Even one day in the office can make me feel like screaming – because I just sit there. I just *sit*! I have to get out. I'm like a border collie, I need walking all the time. Need stimulation. Need natural things bleating at me rather than phones.

And I think humans more and more are realising that we are caging ourselves in the name of safety and security, and we need to get out and explore the natural world even if we've tamed bits of it.

You see, that is why Claire's my trail running guru. And she doesn't just talk a good game. She's rarely out of the mountains or fells, and barely a weekend goes by without her popping up at some trail race or other to film, interview or compete (or sometimes all three). And every morning, the first thing she does, whatever the season, is head outside.

I get up, and I put on my running gear (you should always be prepared for a run in my opinion). I feel really restricted if I ever wear corporate clothes, like I couldn't just break into a cartwheel whenever I wanted to. And before I do anything else – eat breakfast or anything – I just go out. Whatever kind of day it is. Whatever mood the world is in – whether it's a blue sky and it's already happy, or it's raining and lashing down – I always go for a walk, and I always come back feeling refreshed and awake and alive and ready to attack the day. It gives me the energy to sit in front of the computer all day. It's weird. It's my cup of coffee.

I feel more tired at the end of a day sat in front of the computer than I do after running around the Lake District for hours. My brain is just so tired, so fogged up at the end of every day that I kind of need to run just to make it function and get the ideas flowing again. You get your best ideas when you are running on the trails.

It's being in nature that really does it for me. I can run around that field and get 15 ideas in the morning. Running brings the high quicker than walking. And it gives you space. And the thing I really love is feeling the wind on my face. It's like, 'Wow, this is really real! I'm not just in front of a computer typing things, or on the phone.'

And you notice things: you hear the birds, you see the green and the blue and the seasons, you see the trees, you see rabbits running around, and the scenery and the views from a hillside. It just gives you that perspective on life. And reminds you that humans are really animals, but we cage ourselves in these offices and forget that we need to move our bodies and stimulate our brains in different ways.

The freedom is the best thing about trail running. But there's also the camaraderie, the friendships. And you go and run in a new place, you can explore different trails and find new areas, new views, new wildlife. It's the best way to see the world as well.

Claire's spot on about how having a run can make you feel like a new person. The latest research from neuroscientists shows that new neurons are produced in the brain throughout the lifespan – but only one activity is known to trigger the birth of those new neurons: vigorous aerobic exercise. Literally: new run, new you.

And the longer you do it, the bigger the benefits. Even when it hurts. You discover your physical and emotional limitations. And in doing so, you peel back the layers and return to the core of who you are. It's an oft repeated truism, but you genuinely do find out about yourself.

But are we mad to want to do it? Being drawn to these epic events that strip us bare and yet fill us with inner strength? Perhaps the person best placed to answer these questions, with his addiction-riddled past, is Charlie Engle.

You know anybody who finds the need to run a hundred miles or run across a country is in a positive search for more information about themselves. And whether they're trying to fill a gap that's been missing in their life or replacing something that was there before, which was the case for me, I think the beauty of endurance running is that it's a seeker's paradise. It's a sure-fire way to get more information about how you tick. And the more information you have the more likely you are to have better mental health.

Ultra-running – despite its forbidding name – is strangely a lot more accessible than people think. I'm frequently more nervous on the start line of a marathon, or even a 10K, because I know how much it's going to hurt, cardio-wise. Plus there's that pressure to achieve a certain time, especially if you've been training for it. Back to Claire, who spends almost every weekend around endurance races.

It's a lot easier than you think to go and do an ultra-run because it's so slow. It's expected to be slow. You're also expected to stop at checkpoints and chat to the marshals and eat a sandwich and a flapjack. And whatever people's preconceptions, there are a lot of ultra-runners who are a little overweight. They just jog along and it's not very hard to train for a long distance – if you just do plodding. It's actually very pleasant to simply plod along. I loved getting to the fitness level where I could easily plod along for 10 hours. It feels brilliant, it's like going for a walk at that stage of fitness. You're not rushed, you're not stressed, you're not guzzling weird gels and shoving odd-shaped cubes of sugar into your mouth.

She's right about that. I only tend to take gels when I'm running a road marathon and worrying about my time (which is pretty much during all road marathons), and for the rest of the day it'll feel like sumo wrestling in my stomach. Running on trails, just generally, feels more natural.

Even though ultra-running may sound daunting, it really isn't. Not if you build up to it sensibly. And when you're out in the woods, along cliff tops, in mountains, by a river, it somehow feels like you're doing right by your DNA. It's a simplified way of living, almost a sixth sense – going back in time, being unplugged, moving your body, becoming more in tune. And when you run long distances, you feel like you're rediscovering an essential part of yourself, an intuition, an adaptability.

Pheidippides made the epic journey from Athens to Sparta 2,500 years ago in a bid to preserve the new ideals of freedom and democracy, ideals we still hold dear today. Those ancient Greeks built the foundations of Western society. But they also revered their long distance runners, their messengers.

On his way back from Sparta, on the mountain, Pheidippides met the god Pan, who demanded Athenians take more notice of him. *Look after me*, said Pan, *and I'll look after you*. Which they did (they built Pan a temple) and he did (they crushed the invading Persians). Mother Nature might just as well have the same message for us today.

But Pheidippides essentially failed in his mission. He reached Sparta astonishingly quickly but Sparta said no. So he had to run home again to deliver the bad news. Thence to Marathon, where the Greeks attacked anyway, even without Spartan help, and pulled off one of the great military victories. His final journey back to Athens, the one that gave birth to the modern marathon, is the one that did for him.

Pheidippides ran more than 350 miles in a matter of days, but essentially accomplished nothing. And yet we still celebrate him, both the millions who run marathons every year and the joyful few who get to experience the Spartathlon. After all, it's the journey, not the destination.

finishing line

A letter from a volunteer to the 2017 Spartathletes:

Dear Spartathlete,

I am taking the opportunity to write this as I won't be able to be alongside your journey this year. After 13 years of education, it is now time to proceed to university. I'm both nervous and excited, but simultaneously gutted as my course starts before the Spartathlon.

This race is so important and valuable in a multitude of dimensions. A race which only a few are brave enough to attempt, and even fewer are able to conquer. However, this is what's so magical and captivating: the feelings, thoughts, emotions, visions, support, compassion, pain, surprise and doubt one experiences throughout the course. For most athletes participating, the Spartathlon is the highlight of their year, what they've been working for relentlessly. I must admit that it has always been the highlight of my year. I started volunteering when I was 14, at the mountain base, checkpoint 47. I was the young girl thrilled to be providing the runners with their gear, helping them sort everything out quickly and efficiently in order for them to face the dreaded mountain.

I'll never forget what I saw that day, the athletes I met and above all the emotions I felt. It is hard to put into words. I felt so proud of each runner, as if I'd known them and supported their mission throughout. The unforgettable feeling when you're actually of great help to a runner during their unique journey. Such an experience allowed me to develop a passion, which grew stronger and stronger each year. The power of the human body, the workload on each muscle, including the brain. The attitude and aptitude of these athletes. Multiple elements play a fundamental role in ultra-marathons, and it sparked the idea of studying sport and exercise science.

Years later, after having witnessed a lot and seen old and new athletes conquer what to my eyes is mesmerising, I am ready to leave Greece to start my studies in this field. September marks the start of most academic courses, but for me September was always linked to the Spartathlon. Despite the joy and satisfaction it gives me to help athletes who I truly admire, it was my motivating force for the year ahead. This race and the people involved motivate me to become a better person with stronger ambitions, to believe in my efforts, not to succumb to doubt, and above all to work humbly towards something you may not have thought you were capable of.

As three-time champion Szilvia Lubics said, we must each find our own Spartathlon, a goal for which you can work every day. This reminded me of Cavafy's poem 'Ithaca'. In the effort to reach that goal, we must live life, enjoy the journey, and not just simply exist.

To each runner who has participated in the Spartathlon, thank you. Thank you for showing us what humans are capable of, what the body can undergo, the power of the mind to overcome every obstacle, and most importantly, your dedication which in turn leads you to taking a step into these 246km. Even more so, being Greek, the significance of the race is very important. Witnessing athletes from across the world follow the path of Pheidippides gives me a feeling of pride and satisfaction, as you keep our history alive.

I wish you the best of luck for this year. I wish you patience to endure what is ahead of you, peace of mind to think clearly, and above all health, alongside mental and physical strength.

As the great Yiannis Kouros said, 'Like a tree that grows stronger with more branches and roots, you need to find more and more ways to be inspired.' So, may you blossom during your run and have the strength to motivate yourself, whether that's to run faster, reach the next checkpoint, or in the end to climb the last steps to the feet of King Leonidas.

Take care. I hope to be by your side soon,

– Elena

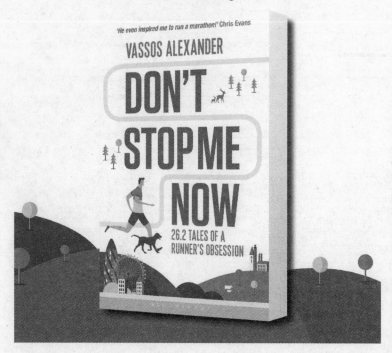